Osseointegration in Dentistry: An Overview
Second Edition

Osseointegration in Dentistry:
An Overview
Second Edition

Edited by

Philip Worthington, MD, BSc

Professor Emeritus and Former Chairman
Department of Oral and Maxillofacial Surgery
University of Washington School of Dentistry
Seattle, Washington

Brien R. Lang, DDS, MS

Professor Emeritus
University of Michigan School of Dentistry
Ann Arbor, Michigan

Jeffrey E. Rubenstein, DMD, MS

Professor and Director
Prosthodontic Faculty Practice and Maxillofacial Prosthetic Service
Department of Prosthodontics
University of Washington School of Dentistry
Seattle, Washington

quintessence books

Quintessence Publishing Co, Inc

Chicago, Berlin, Tokyo, Copenhagen, London, Paris, Milan, Barcelona, Istanbul, São Paulo, New Delhi, Moscow, Prague, and Warsaw

We dedicate this book to those who have taught us what we know, to those who seek to learn, and to our families for their forbearance.

Library of Congress Cataloging-in-Publication Data

Osseointegration in dentistry : an overview / edited by Philip Worthington, Brien R. Lang, Jeffrey E. Rubenstein.— 2nd ed.
      p. ; cm.
Includes bibliographical references and index.
  ISBN 0-86715-425-X (pbk.)
 1. Osseointegrated dental implants. 2. Osseointegration.
  [DNLM: 1. Dental Implantation, Endosseous. 2. Osseointegration. WU
640 O843 2003] I. Worthington, Philip. II. Lang, Brien R. III.
Rubenstein, Jeffrey E.
  RK667.I45O86 2003
  617.6'9—dc21
                               2003013104

©2003 Quintessence Publishing Co, Inc

Quintessence Publishing Co, Inc
4350 Chandler Drive
Hanover Park, IL 60133
www.quintpub.com

Editor: Kathryn O'Malley
Production and Design: Dawn Hartman

Printed in Canada

Table of Contents

Preface to the Second Edition

The concept of osseointegration and its application to dental practice were introduced into North America at the beginning of the 1980s. Since then, many changes have taken place, not in the basic theory and to only a limited extent in surgical technique, but predominantly in the refinement and sophistication of the prosthodontic or dental restorative phase of treatment. The original edition of this book—entitled *Osseointegration in Dentistry: An Introduction*—has now been revised and expanded with the intention of providing the reader with insight into the developments that have taken place on the basis of further experiments and clinical experience.

It remains the intention of the editors to direct this book to the dental student, as well as to the practicing dentist, who wishes to understand the place of osseointegration in the overall scheme of oral reconstruction. Many chapters have been rewritten and other sections have been added to address previously neglected topics such as the placement of implants in the esthetic zone, variations in abutment design, and the role of osseointegrated implants in more advanced procedures. The student is again advised to follow a path of stepwise learning, proceeding from the simpler to the more complex.

Preface to the First Edition

This text is intended to introduce the reader to the concept of osseointegration and its place in modern dental practice. It is a primer, not a technical manual, and it is hoped that it will serve to orient the beginner to the profound impact that osseointegration has had on clinical dentistry.

Basic concepts are presented and the place of osseointegration in the overall scheme of dental treatment planning is illustrated. The reader will come to realize that osseointegration refers not to a development in technique but to a fundamental biologic phenomenon with far-reaching applications throughout the fields of medicine and dentistry. Its importance is difficult to overestimate, but most would agree that it is one of the most significant advances in dentistry in the last half century. This book is aimed at dental students who need a simple introduction to the topic while familiarizing themselves with traditional patterns of dental treatment, and at dental practitioners who are beginning to study osseointegration and its applications. For further study, it is anticipated that readers will progress to more advanced texts such as *Tissue-Integrated Prostheses*, edited by Brånemark, Zarb, and Albrektsson (Quintessence, 1985), and *Advanced Osseointegration Surgery*, edited by Worthington and Brånemark (Quintessence, 1992).

Contributors

Michael R. Arcuri, DDS, MS
Private Practice
Cedar Falls, Iowa

John B. Brunski, MS, PhD
Professor
Department of Biomedical Engineering
Rensselaer Polytechnic Institute
Troy, New York

Lars G. Hollender, DDS
Professor and Director of Oral Radiology
Department of Oral Medicine
University of Washington School of
    Dentistry
Seattle, Washington

Brien R. Lang, DDS, MS
Professor Emeritus
University of Michigan School of Dentistry
Ann Arbor, Michigan

Robert B. O'Neal, DMD, MS, MEd
Associate Professor
Department of Periodontics
University of Washington School of
    Dentistry
Seattle, Washington

Michael E. Razzoog, DDS, MS, MPH
Professor
Biologic and Materials Sciences
Division of Prosthodontics
University of Michigan School of Dentistry
Ann Arbor, Michigan

Jeffrey E. Rubenstein, DMD, MS
Professor and Director
Prosthodontic Faculty Practice and
    Maxillofacial Prosthetic Service
Department of Prosthodontics
University of Washington School of
    Dentistry
Seattle, Washington

Clark M. Stanford, DDS, PhD
Centennial Fund Professor
Dows Institute for Dental Research
University of Iowa College of Dentistry
Iowa City, Iowa

Philip Worthington, MD, BSc
Professor Emeritus and Former Chairman
Department of Oral and Maxillofacial
    Surgery
University of Washington School of
    Dentistry
Seattle, Washington

chapter 1

Introduction

Philip Worthington, MD, BSc

History of Implants

Since tooth loss from disease and trauma has always been a feature of humankind's existence, it is not surprising that the history of tooth replacement is a long one. Evidence from ancient civilizations shows that attempts were made to replace missing teeth by banding artificial tooth replacements to remaining teeth with metal many centuries ago.

There are two elements in tooth replacement: material for the replacement of teeth, and some form of attachment mechanism. Throughout the ages, and particularly during this century, great ingenuity has been devoted to both these components. Various materials have been used for replacement teeth, including carved ivory and bone. At times, natural teeth extracted from the poor have been used to provide replacements for the missing teeth of the wealthy. In more recent times, porcelain and plastic have provided most of the replacement units.

As for the mechanism of attachment, clinicians have long sought an analog for the periodontal ligament. Experiments were made, sometimes by the unscrupulous on the unsuspecting, in vain attempts to develop a fibrous attachment that could serve the same purposes as the periodontal ligament. The latter is, however, a specialized structure that serves not only as an efficient attachment mechanism but also as a shock absorber and a sensory organ. Furthermore, it is capable of mediating bony remodeling and allowing tooth movement. Easy to underestimate, it is impossible to reproduce. The search for an artificial periodontal ligament has proven fruitless and misguided.

Implants may indeed be anchored in bone by means of a surrounding sheath of connective tissue, but in general this has not shown the degree of organization and specialization that would allow it to pass as a substitute for a periodontal ligament. In most cases, loading leads to gradual widening of the fibrous tissue layer and loosening of the implant, with consequent implant failure. In contrast to the periodontal ligament, a fibrous tissue sheath is a poorly differentiated layer of scar tissue.

An alternative attachment mechanism was discovered, by means of an accidental finding, during experimental work carried out in Sweden by Professor Per-Ingvar Brånemark and his colleagues during the 1950s and 1960s. Brånemark was a physician—not a dentist—with an interest in the microcirculation of bone and the problems of wound healing. He studied these by means of vital microscopy, a technique whereby a thin layer of living tissue is prepared and examined under the microscope. To facilitate this, he used an implantable optical device housed in metal and placed surgically into the bone of the experimental animal. This observation chamber allowed light to be transmitted through the thin tissue layer; circulatory and cellular changes could thus be observed in the living tissue. This technique was not new. Similar observation chambers had been used by other researchers. What became significant, however, was that when the metal titanium was used for the observation chamber and the device was introduced into the bone with a gentle surgical technique, the bone was found to adhere to the metal with great tenacity.

The metallic structure became incorporated in the living bone in a way formerly believed to be impossible. Brånemark realized the significance of this new form of attachment mechanism, not merely for dental implant purposes but for orthopedic uses, too, and he called it *osseointegration*. He then set about studying the phenomenon in great detail.

Certain circumstances are necessary for titanium to become rigidly incorporated into living bone. The titanium surface must not be merely clean or even sterile; it must be free from contamination and in a reactive state. The bony implant bed must be prepared with great gentleness, inflicting minimal damage to the tissue. Close congruency of the metallic item and the bone is important. To maximize the chances of successful osseointegration, a period of undisturbed healing time is desirable to allow the bone to grow up to and fuse with the layer of oxides on the implant surface. If all the desirable circumstances are present, then osseointegration of this unique metal takes place—predictably—in a high percentage of cases.

Prior to the Brånemark era, many ingenious clinicians had worked with many designs of implantable devices intended to support a dental superstructure. These included frameworks resting on the jaw but beneath the mucoperiosteum; frameworks that had bony contact only at the mandibular symphysis and at the ascending rami, but which were otherwise supramucosal; and a wide variety of intraosseous devices of varying shapes and sizes. Some of these could function well over many years, and they kept hope alive for the developing field of implantology. Others failed at varying rates and tended to gain a bad reputation. In these early implants, predictability was lacking.

The significance of the Brånemark work is that it stressed the need to understand biology, to use the natural healing processes of the body when introducing a metallic foreign body into the bone. The prepared implant site was viewed, correctly, as a wound—a wound in which tissue injury had to be minimized. The special characteristics of titanium were important, particularly its resistance to corrosion and its biocompatibility. It seems that when the necessary conditions are present, living bone has difficulty in recognizing that titanium is a foreign substance.

The successful osseointegrated implant is therefore one in which there is a direct connection between living bone and titanium. This attachment must, and can, endure under conditions of loading. There is no fibrous tissue sheath surrounding the implant; hence the osseointegrated implant is more akin to an ankylosed tooth root than a normal tooth root.

What Is Osseointegration?

Osseointegration is a biologic concept. It refers to the incorporation within living bone of an inanimate (metallic) component. It is in essence an anchorage mechanism—nothing more, nothing less. Such anchorage allows the attachment of prosthetic components to the skeleton by means of these anchorage units. The success of osseointegration has been proven beyond all doubt, but successful achievement of osseointegration depends on careful planning, meticulous surgical technique, and skillful prosthetic management. It demands an appreciation for biology and an understanding of wound healing in particular. Its applications are wide ranging, including not only dental prostheses but maxillofacial prostheses, replacement of diseased joints, and the attachment of artificial limbs. The chapters that follow provide a better understanding of this fascinating biologic phenomenon.

Types of Dental Implants

There are now so many proprietary brands of implants available that it is not feasible to survey them all in this introductory text.

The student should be aware, however, of the ways in which dental implants may be classified and must understand the general categories into which they fit. Implants may be classified according to their position, their constituent material, and their morphologic design.

Position

Implants may be *subperiosteal, transosseous,* or *endosseous.*

Subperiosteal implants

Subperiosteal implants consist of a non-osseointegrated framework that rests on the surface of the jaw (Fig 1-1). It can be used for either the maxilla or the mandible, although most subperiosteal implants are mandibular. Subperiosteal implants are usually bilateral, but they can be unilateral. The framework rests beneath the mucoperiosteum, with posts that penetrate the mucosa into the mouth, usually supporting an overdenture. Some of these implants have served patients well for many years, but even the best series have shown marked failure rates after 10 years, and many more have lasted for much shorter periods. Problems have included infection, exteriorization by downgrowth of epithelium, and damage to the underlying bone. Removal may also be difficult.

Transosseous implants

The most common form of transosseous implant is the transmandibular staple, which has a plate that fits against the lower border of the mandible at the symphysis and has posts rising from it (Fig 1-2). Some of these posts pass into the jaw and others pass through it into the mouth, where they serve to stabilize a denture. Some are made

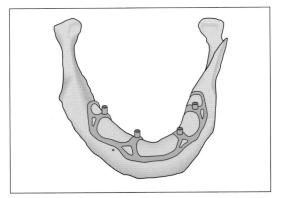

Fig 1-1 Subperiosteal implants are custom-cast frameworks supported by the mandible.

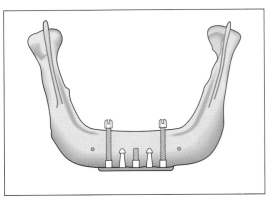

Fig 1-2 The mandibular staple bone plate is an exemplary form of transosseous implant.

of vitallium, some of titanium alloy, and some of gold alloy. Transosseous implants are introduced through a submental incision, usually under general anesthesia in a hospital setting. They are used only for the mandible. Bone loss around the posts has proved a frequent problem.

Endosseous implants

Endosseous implants are placed into the maxilla or mandible through intraoral incisions in the mucoperiosteum (Fig 1-3). The shapes and construction materials vary. Endosseous implants are the most commonly used implant type, and this is the fastest growing part of the dental implant market. They may be used for single-tooth replacement, partially edentulous jaws, and totally edentulous jaws. Most claim to be osseointegrated.

Materials

Many materials have been used for implants, including ceramics such as aluminum oxide and metals ranging from al-

loys of gold, titanium, and nickel-chrome-vanadium to commercially pure titanium.

Designs

Many endosseous implants conform more or less to the shape of a tooth root, being either in the form of a tapered cylinder or a true cylinder. Some have threads on the external surface, and others do not (see Fig 1-3). Some are solid screws. Some have external fins rather than threads. Some are hollow cylinders with fenestrations, called *baskets*. Still others are flat plates, called *blades* (see Fig 1-3). Many of these endosseous implants are made of commercially pure titanium or a titanium alloy, and some are finished with a titanium plasma-sprayed surface. Others have a coating of hydroxyapatite, a porous ceramic bone substitute, which may allow the ingrowth of living bone and hence improve anchorage.

The clinician may easily be bewildered by the variety of implants available. In making a selection of one or more implant systems for use, it is important to remember

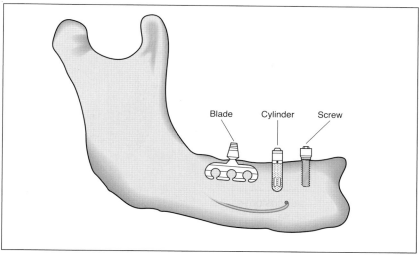

Fig 1-3 Endosseous implant designs are varied. The more recent cylinder and screw types are more successful than blade types.

to view all manufacturers' claims with healthy skepticism. A survey of practicing dentists provided the following list of features thought important in making a choice of implant system:

- Demonstrated reliability (over at least 5 years)
- American Dental Association approval
- Quality of instrumentation
- Quality of prosthodontics
- Versatility
- Reputation of the manufacturing company
- Ease of use
- Training and after-sales service
- Cost to the patient
- Start-up cost

In evaluating an implant system, the clinician may well ask the following:

- Were animal experiments conducted before the product was marketed?
- Were prospective clinical trials undertaken?
- Are the results of at least 5-year-long trials published in reputable journals?
- Have there been multicenter replication studies?

The practitioner should realize that it is not valid to extrapolate results from one product to another merely on the basis of some superficial morphologic resemblance. The composition of the material, its purity, its surface characteristics, and its preparation are of vital importance. Furthermore, the reports of implant trials should state clearly the criteria used for judging success, and studies should report all implants consecutively placed, not merely selected cases.

chapter 2

Biocompatibility, Tissue Responses, and Concepts of the Implant Interface

Clark M. Stanford, DDS, PhD

From the time of their introduction to North America in the early 1980s, the use of endosseous dental implants for the support of dental crowns and dentures has led to a revolution in the routine approach to dental care. Prior to this era, numerous implant designs and clinical procedures were used that often resulted in significant side effects of infection, implant fracture, and/or unpredictable outcomes. In addition, clinical outcomes of care were often poorly documented in the dental literature (eg, opinionated, anecdotal case reports), in which elaborate but unsubstantiated claims were made about the benefits of each implant system. Starting in the early 1960s, investigative teams in Sweden and Switzerland began programs to rigorously evaluate implant designs and devise surgical protocols for the predictable placement and restoration of dental implants. Prior to the introduction of this new implant design and specific surgical protocols to North America in 1982, there were serial case reports and controlled clinical trials with a common se-

ries of documented outcome measures that demonstrated for the first time that screw-type dental implants could be placed predictably into the anterior mandible of patients. Using careful surgical procedures in which the amount of heat generated was limited (because heat causes cell death and an excessive loss of blood supply to the surrounding bone), one was able to place titanium implants into bone and achieve a significant amount of direct bone contact between living cortical and cancellous bone and the oxide surface of the implant, a concept referred to as *osseointegration* (Fig 2-1). Over a series of studies subsequently performed, it is now known that the high clinical success rates (greater than 95%) for this procedure occur by way of initial implant stability provided by the amount, quality, and distribution of bone within the proposed implant site. This has led to the expanded use of dental implants in multiple areas of the mouth (ie, replacement of single teeth and partially edentulous spans as well as completely edentulous jaws). It is

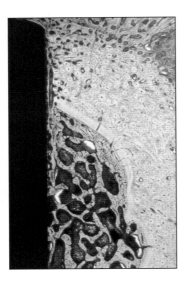

Fig 2-1 Cortical and cancellous bone contact occurs along the implant interface in a process known as *osseointegration*.

safe to say that implant treatment has now become the standard of care for replacement of missing teeth, rather than an experimental treatment waiting to be proven.

One clinical limitation in evaluating implant outcomes has been a lack of quantitative measurement approaches that can be used to evaluate the relative status of an implant. Currently, these relatively crude clinical parameters include a lack of signs or symptoms of pathology, a lack of mobility, and a radiographic assessment of the interface. The clinical success of implants relies on both short-term surgical issues (adequate bone volume, minimal surgical trauma, etc) and long-term biologic responses through masticatory load–mediated bone adaptation to the implant.[1] This long-term response is only achieved through dynamic modeling (a net change in bone shape) and remodeling (the continuous turnover of bone with-

out a net change in shape or size) processes of bone (see Stanford and Brand[1]). This adaptive biologic capacity allows bone to withstand the tolerances of clinical function (eg, the inaccuracy of technical procedures and masticatory loading parameters), while creating essentially a structural material capable of supporting clinical loads over long periods of time. While high success rates hold for certain anatomic regions, the bony response within the thin cortical plates and diminished cancellous bone characterized as Type 4 bone by Lekholm and Zarb is considerably less successful with conventional machined-surface implants (ie, 65% to 85%).[2] For instance, in a systematic review of a series of clinical trials appearing in the dental literature (referred to as a meta-analysis), Lindh et al observed that implant success in the posterior maxilla is lower than that of other regions of the mouth and is highly dependent on adequate bone volume in the area.[3] For these reasons, the response of trabecular bone to the mechanical environment is a critical factor, especially in the edentulous posterior maxilla. Multiple strategies have also been proposed to increase the local quantity and quality of osseous tissue at the interface to boost the predictability of implant therapy for patients with poor bone quality, as well as to allow for modifications of the conventional surgical protocols (eg, immediate loading) that assist patients in enjoying the benefits of predictable implant therapy.

To increase the predictability of implant therapy, significant efforts have gone into development of implant biomaterials that hold the promise of improving clinical success. Unfortunately, the dental implant market is currently being driven by the perceived need for biomaterial "innovations," while sometimes the real need is purely market position. It is important that the clinician understand that even though there are more than 60 implant systems on the market in the United States, there is no requirement that they document any clinical success (or survival). The US Food and Drug Administration simply requires a few mechanical tests of the new implant and assurance of good manufacturing practices (GMPs) to allow marketing of a new dental implant. The first clinical trial therefore often takes place in the dental office. The purpose of this chapter is to provide a framework and background for the clinician to understand the basic processes in implant healing and to discuss the relative merits of various clinical and laboratory means to evaluate the biologic response to the implant surface.

Biocompatibility

When biologic tissues such as bone and other connective tissues interact with inorganic metals, a variety of responses can occur. These reactions vary from highly reactive pathologic processes, including the formation of corrosion products from metals such as stainless steel, to passive reactions on metal surfaces possessing a highly reactive surface energy with oxygen. These latter types of metal form what are known as *passivated surface oxides*.[4] These oxides form a relatively stable layer on the surface of certain metals when metal ions (M) interact thermodynamically with oxygen, forming stable oxide species (MO_x). There are many metals that form surface oxides, such as aluminum, chrome-cobalt, and nickel-chrome. Most of these, however, are not useful as long-term biomaterials because corrosion of the metals leads to a continuous release of metallic ions into the surrounding tissues. Acute and chronic localized inflammatory responses (eg, Type IV) can result in the eventual encapsulation of the implant in a fibrous capsule (ie, *marsupialization*) as the body attempts to wall off the offensive material from itself.

Titanium is a common, lightweight, non-noble metal that is corrosion resistant as the result of the formation of a surface oxide. Because of these properties, titanium is often used in ship and airplane construction and is a useful material in the human body. Titanium's tenacious surface oxide (primarily titanium dioxide, TiO_2), provides a stable interface on which mineralizing bone matrix can be deposited. This oxide surface provides an initial 50- to 100-Å-thick surface that becomes coated by blood-derived plasma proteins (especially fibronectin and

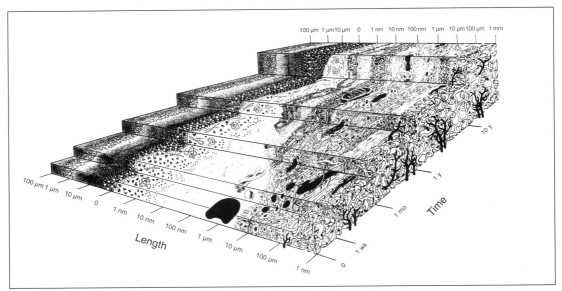

Fig 2-2 The process of osseointegration is an ongoing process that starts with an initial blood clot and over time ends with mature bone around the implant. The healing process is logarithmic, with initial healing occurring in the first month, followed by tissue maturation through the first year following placement. (Reprinted with permission from Kasemo and Lausmaa.[5])

vitronectin) at the time of implant placement. It is from the biologic inertness of this oxide surface that implants derive the important property of *biocompatibility* (essentially a process where the body simply does not respond to the metal but recognizes it immunologically as *self*).

Observation of a clinically loaded dental implant reveals a fascinating series of changes. Six years after placement, the passivated titanium oxide layer has grown in thickness from the initial 50 to 100 Å to approximately 2,000 Å. When the composition of the newly formed oxide is evaluated, it is found to contain organic and inorganic materials (calcium, phosphorus, and sulfur), suggesting that the implant's surface oxide is reactive and interacts with the body in a dynamic and ongoing process of integration (Fig 2-2). When pure titanium or titanium alloy (Ti-6Al-4V) surfaces are initially exposed to physiologic blood, a complex of titanium-phosphate and calcium-containing hydroxyl groups spontaneously forms on the oxide surface, indicating that titanium reacts with water, mineral ions, and plasma fluids from the time of placement. The oxide surface also plays a role, along with bone remodeling, in creating an adaptive interfacial region rather than simply a sharply demarcated boundary between the implant and the body. Thus, the reactive nature of this oxide surface, with its spontaneous formation of a calcium-phosphate apatite, is one reason why titanium appears to be so biocompatible.

Healing Responses

Since the healing response of bone creates the formation of a complex mineralizing matrix, the healing response of the biologic tissues and the oxide surface is really a two-phase interaction between the newly forming hydroxyapatite bone matrix and the surface oxide (also a form of ceramic). In turn, the thickness, composition, and (potentially) the reactive nature of the implant's ceramic oxide are sensitive to the way in which the surface of the implant is cleaned and sterilized by the manufacturer. The cleaning and handling procedures for implants, which include scrupulous surface cleaning in a controlled environment and minimal handling by the operator prior to the time of placement, are therefore very important. In addition to the surface contaminants, a number of other physical and chemical features of the oxide layer will influence biologic responses to implants. These features include the surface chemistry (oxide composition and thickness), surface energy, and surface topography (size, shape, roughness, etc).

When an implant is placed into a prepared site, the ability of the body to respond to the "trauma" induced by this procedure will influence the tissue response (and hence the degree of integration). Proper surgical handling of the tissues, with minimal generation of heat (below 47°C for 1 minute or less) during preparation of the surgical site (osteotomy) and careful handling of the soft tissues, will provide a predictable long-term result. Following formation of the initial clot around the surgical site, a minor inflammatory response occurs, with the proliferation and differentiation of phagocytes and undifferentiated mesenchymal cells from the adjacent periosteum and wall

of the osteotomy (appositional growth). The ability of tissues to differentiate depends on the presence of intact vascular beds. In turn, a poor blood supply leads to an oxygen-poor environment that stimulates proliferation of fibrous and cartilaginous tissues instead of mineralization of bone.

Following placement of the implant, a thin (about 0.5- to 1.0-mm) layer of peri-implant bone in the prepared site will become necrotic (composed of dead and dying cells) simply from the process of forming the implant site. The body must replace this bone as integration proceeds. Initially, an ingrowth of vascular loops occurs at a rate of 0.5 mm per day, followed by formation of a loose, collagenous cell–rich matrix in the first 4 weeks after initial surgical implant placement. Due to the inert nature of the oxide surface, newly differentiating osteoblastic cells derived from the adjacent periosteum will synthesize a woven bone matrix that provides initial bone contact with the oxide surface. Following this initial contact, a remodeling phase is initiated by week 4, in which hematopoietic-derived osteoclastic cells remove the established woven matrix (at a rate of 40 μm per day). Following the resorptive process (a coordinated process in which osteoclasts and osteoblasts interact), an osteogenic front of lamellar bone differentiation occurs, with newly differentiated osteoblasts laying down a mature Haversian bone system in a process that is influenced by environmental factors such as micromovements of the interface, local vascular supply, and systemic and local release of matrix-regulating growth factors (for further information, see the review by Stanford and Brand[1]).

The initial healing processes have been studied in optical healing chambers in which a fibrovascular tissue is observed to grow into the region of the screw threads (at the phenomenal rate of 85.5 μm per day), peaking around the third week following implant placement.[6] Under an electron microscope, this growing interface exhibits a relationship demonstrating an intimate contact between the extracellular matrix formed by maturing osteoblastic cells and the titanium oxide surface. The actual contact between bone and the oxide surface is composed of a rich layer of a specific set of bone matrix proteins (osteopontin and bone sialoprotein) and small, lipid-rich proteins called biglycan and decorin.[7,8] These proteins are proposed to act as molecular "glue" to bond the matrix to the implant surface (similar to their role in gluing layers of bone together in the histologically described "cement" lines of mature bone).

Implant Retentive Features

When implants are placed into the jaw, two stages of osseointegration occur. *Primary integration* is the process of initial wound healing that is assured through maintenance of a nonmobile (fixation) contact between the osteotomy and the implant. In time, the initial bone contact is turned over as a function of *secondary osseointegration*. To ensure rigid initial fixation (ie, *primary osseointegration*), implants use a series of three major macro-retentive features on their surface: screw threads (tapped or self-tapping), solid-body press-fit designs, and/or sintered bead technologies. Prevention of movement (*micromovement*) greater than 100 μm is critical to prevent the formation of fibrous tissue around the implant body. An important biologic principle of bone is that it responds favorably to compressive loading (without the presence of a periodontal ligament) but not to shear forces.[1] Therefore, these macroscopic designs act to achieve compressive loading of the surrounding cortical and cancellous bone. These design innovations have included rounded thread tips, angled pitches, and multiple thread-cutting profiles (with or without a screw-based press-fit), where two or more sets of threads are cut at different relative locations in the osteotomy as a means to reduce initial stripping (eg, upon overseating) and consequent loss of primary osseointegration.

The process of *secondary integration* is primarily dependent on the pattern of replacement of the initial bone contact with mature, load-carrying bone around the implant surface. The ability to both assist primary osseointegration and direct secondary osseointegration by way of altering the surface of the titanium implant has been one of the most significant innovations since the introduction of the original, smooth, machined-surface implants. These strategies can be divided into those that attempt to enhance the in-migration of new bone, a process known as *osteoconduction*, through changes in surface topography (eg, surface "roughness"). Second are biologic approaches to manipulate the types of cells that grow onto the surface and strategies to use the implant as a vehicle for local delivery of a bioactive coating (adhesion matrix or growth factor such as bone morphogenetic protein). Ideally, this would lead to *osteoinduction* of new bone differentiation along the implant surface. At the current time, alterations of surface roughness have been the primary means used to manipulate the healing process in commercially available implant systems.

Implant Micro-retentive Features: A Role for Surface Roughness

Various implant surfaces have been created though sandblasting or grit-blasting of the surface, sometimes followed by an acid-etching procedure. These various surface treatments are aimed at increasing the available surface area on the metal. This enhanced surface area then allows a greater area for load transfer of bone against the implant surface. The ability to define what surface roughness actually is has led to some controversy in the literature, since roughness is often difficult to define (it is operationally defined by the measurement approach one chooses to define it, and it varies across the surface of the implant, eg, the roughness is different at screw tips versus at the base of the thread profile). A number of investigators have theoretically and experimentally defined an optimal surface roughness as the presence of surface pits or holes of 1.5 to 5 µm on the surface of the implant.[9,10] These micromechanical surface features in turn influence the process of secondary osseointegration.[1,11] An additional advantage of acid etching or electrochemical oxide growth is to increase the roughness of the grit-blasted surface as well as clean and remove residual grit from the implant surface.

Clinical Measurement of Osseointegration

The clinician often asks the puzzling question, "When can I safely restore this implant and provide clinical function for my patient?" There really is no single answer, but a number of measurement approaches can be used.

A common research method to evaluate implant healing is to measure the extent of bone contact along the implant surface that can be assessed at the light microscopic level (referred to as *histomorphometry*). In this approach, an implant is removed from an experimental animal with the surrounding bone, and thin sections are made that can be viewed under the microscope. Various measurements can then be made, such as the percentage of bone contact and thread fill. Often the degree of contact is then compared to the relative strength of the bone contact by attempting to remove the implant destructively in a materials testing machine. In research studies, another measurement technique involves placement of a torque driver on the implant and application of an unscrewing force (reverse torque test) until the implant-bone contact is clinically ruptured. Values for this approach for an otherwise clinically healthy implant vary from 50 to 70 Ncm.[12,13] Some clinicians use a similar approach in patients with a reverse (counterclockwise) torque, which is used to evaluate whether the implant can be clinically loaded. The drawbacks to this approach include the inability to know before one performs such a procedure if the implant interface is simply immature (and rupturing it will unnecessarily delay or inhibit integration) and the fact that it is an uncontrolled and catastrophic test (which is consequently expensive for both the clinician and patient). While it is unclear at the present time how much bone contact is needed for an implant to remain clinically stable in the long term, it does appear that the following are consistently true. The amount of bony contact

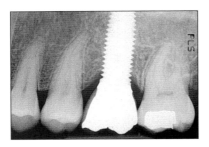

Fig 2-3 Radiographs provide clinical information about the proximal bone heights but little information about the status of bone on the facial or lingual aspects.

around an implant will vary between 30% and 70%, with a common average around 50% contact.[1] The amount of contact can vary significantly, depending on where the measurement is made on any one implant, and the degree of bone contact will change with ongoing bone remodeling. The strategic role of surface topography in this process is to accelerate the formation of bone contact and to maintain this contact over time. This allows implant therapy to be used in a more accelerated fashion than previously thought, as well as provide applications to anatomic areas (eg, the posterior maxilla) previously thought to be at greater risk for implant failures.

From the perspective of clinical reality, the clinician needs a routine method to determine whether osseointegration has taken place. Conventionally, implant success criteria has depended on the use of a series of crude clinical assessments: Does the implant move when manipulated between two instruments? Are there signs of peri-implant radiolucency? Are there signs of infection or pain? For a 21st-century treatment modality, it seems odd to use 18th-century means to assess the health of an implant. To this end, there have been a number of measurement approaches developed to allow the clinician

to assess the health of an implant. One currently available approach is to assess the degree of torque needed during the drilling and implant placement steps. To do this, the surgeon uses a special drill with a built-in torque load cell that provides a readout of the resistance given by the bone during the drilling process. Logically, the thick cortical bone in the anterior mandible will provide a high level of resistance to drilling and implant placement (greater primary osseointegration), in comparison to the thin cortical plates and poor trabeculation of the posterior maxilla. While this approach is useful at the time of implant placement, it provides little useful information 3 to 6 months later, when the restorative dentist is trying to decide whether it is safe to put the implant into clinical function.

Of the various conventional techniques used to measure implant integration, the use of standardized parallel radiographic images has been considered the most reliable. Radiographs, especially periapical and computerized tomographic images, provide valuable information for treatment planning. Realistically, though, they are only a relative (mesial and distal) measurement of bone contact against the side of a clinically functioning implant; significant bony changes can occur on the facial and lingual aspects of the implant, which are missed by conventional radiography (Fig 2-3). The major limitations of this approach are technique sensitivity, which results in numerous errors (eg, errors in the angle of the central beam relative to the film, processing errors, human interpretation), as well as difficulty in evaluating the exact changes in bone quality (bone density) following implant loading along the implant interface. Recent advancements in digital radiography and digital subtraction radiography are a helpful refinement of this approach. Radiography, though, is a form of imaging and will therefore always suffer from a lack of definitive association between the actual amount of bone contact (biologic integration) and the resultant image provided to the clinician.

Conventional clinical tests for implant integration attempt to measure the relative bone contact (and more precisely, the stiffness of this contact) by such crude methods as rapping the head of the implant with a mirror handle (listening for a high-pitched "ring," indicative of bony contact, versus a dull "thud," indicative of fibrous tissue encapsulation). While this may seem absurdly crude, the basis behind this approach is actually very important. Impact testing evaluates three types of stiffness around the implant: the implant itself, the interface, and the surrounding bone. In the 1980s, a device was developed for the quantitative measurement of movement to objectively evaluate the periodontal support of teeth. This device (Periotest; Gulden Medizintechnik, Bensheim, Germany) is a small, electrically driven accelerometer that is held against the side of a tooth. A small hammer then strikes the tooth, and the amount of elastic damping of the tooth–periodontal ligament complex is measured on a scale of −8 to +50 Periotest values (PTV). Following its introduction, a number of investigators used the Periotest to evaluate the stability of dental implants. While the device has proven useful for the evaluation of teeth, it is of limited value in the evaluation of implant integration. The primary reason for this is because implants have a very limited lateral range of motion (< 25 μm) versus teeth (125 to 300 μm), resulting in a very limited range of output from the device. Essentially, if the implant is stable, one gets a range of −5 to +5 PTV; if it has failed, one gets an elevated PTV. The actual discriminatory ability of the device to determine whether the implant is healthy is consequently very limited; one can feel the same difference with the fingers with the conventional two-instrument approach. The Periotest measurement is also technique sensitive, since the measurement is dependent on factors such as the angle and position of the striking hammer and the length of the abutment.

While the Periotest (and similar physical-impact testing devices) has proven to be of limited use, the alternative application of high-frequency sonic (acoustic sound) energy to the implant has been shown to be a useful means of measuring the relative implant integration. In this case, the force applied is an order of magnitude lower than the Periotest. Measurement of sonic vibration to an implant is much like listening to a tuning fork after it has been struck. In this case, a small electric transducer applies a small (< 1 μm) swept-wave vibration to the implant, and a second transducer then measures the resulting change in the vibration (Fig 2-4). One device (Osstell; Integration Diagnostics, Sävedalen, Sweden) is currently available for what is known as resonance frequency analysis (RFA). The development,

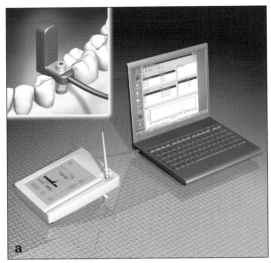
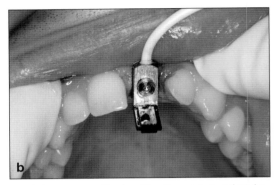

Fig 2-4 Resonance frequency analysis (RFA) is one approach to measure the health of bone around an implant. The technique uses a transducer to apply a vibration to the implant and a second transducer to measure the damping of the signal. In clinical use, the RFA approach can be performed with a computerized approach *(a)* to quickly read the stability of an implant prior to restoration. The transducer is attached to the implant body *(b)* and the measurement made.

background, and validation of this technique for dental implants was established by Dr Neal Meredith. RFA uses two small parallel piezoceramic transducers that are positioned on either the implant or the implant abutment. A computer-based measurement is then made in which an excitation signal of 5 to 15 kHz (peak amplitude 1 V) is applied to the implant, and the first flexural resonance (high-resolution damping) of the signal is measured. While the technology is sophisticated, the computational technology has been simplified to provide a simple and understandable measurement scale. On a standard scale of 1 to 100, the implant stability quotient (ISQ) is rapidly (< 5 seconds) provided to the clinician. This measurement approach has high resolution, reproducibility, and promise as a means to repeatedly evaluate the relative state of implant integration.[14–16] RFA is most valuable in its ability to individualize for each implant how long the healing period must be, versus the common and somewhat arbitrary 3 to 6 months used for delayed loading of implants following placement.

Summary

Implant dentistry has enjoyed an exploding number of new applications, techniques, materials, and devices since the early 1980s. Patient acceptance of implant therapy has resulted from the high success rates of the conventional surgical and restorative protocols. In an effort to increase the predictability of this therapy, there has been an ongoing evolution in implant surface technologies, biomechanics, and understanding of the biology of the implant interface. Clinical dentistry has seen dental implant treatment move from an "experimental" therapy to one that is biologically, clinically, and esthetically predictable. It is the treatment of the 21st century.

References

1. Stanford CM, Brand RA. Toward an understanding of implant occlusion and strain adaptive bone modeling and remodeling. J Prosthet Dent 1999; 81:553–561.
2. Zarb GA, Lewis DW. Dental implants and decision making. J Dent Educ 1992;56:863–872.
3. Lindh T, Gunne J, Tillberg A, Molin M. A meta-analysis of implants in partial edentulism. Clin Oral Implants Res 1998;9:80–90.
4. Stanford CM, Keller JC, Solursh M. Bone cell expression on titanium surfaces is altered by sterilization treatments. J Dent Res 1994;73: 1061–1071.
5. Kasemo B, Lausmaa J. Surface science aspects on inorganic biomaterials. CRC Crit Rev Biocompatibil 1986;2:335–380.
6. Goodman S, Toksvig-Larsen S, Aspenberg P. Ingrowth of bone into pores in titanium chambers implanted in rabbits: Effect of pore cross-sectional shape in the presence of dynamic shear. J Biomed Mater Res 1993;27:247–253.
7. Puleo DA, Nanci A. Understanding and controlling the bone-implant interface. Biomaterials 1999;20:2311–2321.
8. Cooper LF, Yliheikkila PK, Felton DA, Whitson SW. Spatiotemporal assessment of fetal bovine osteoblast culture differentiation indicates a role for BSP in promoting differentiation. J Bone Miner Res 1998;13:620–632.
9. Hansson S. Surface roughness parameters as predictors of anchorage strength in bone: A critical analysis. J Biomech 2000;33:1297–1303.
10. Wennerberg A, Albrektsson T. Suggested guidelines for the topographic evaluation of implant surfaces. Int J Oral Maxillofac Implants 2000;15: 331–344.
11. Stanford CM. Biomechanical and functional behavior of implants. Adv Dent Res 1999;13:88–92.
12. Brånemark R, Ohrnell LO, Nilsson P, Thomsen P. Biomechanical characterization of osseointegration during healing: An experimental in vivo study in the rat. Biomaterials 1997;18:969–978.
13. Baker D, London RM, O'Neal R. Rate of pull-out strength gain of dual-etched titanium implants: A comparative study in rabbits. Int J Oral Maxillofac Implants 1999;14:722–728.
14. Meredith N. A review of nondestructive test methods and their application to measure the stability and osseointegration of bone-anchored endosseous implants. Crit Rev Biomed Eng 1998; 26:275–291.
15. Sennerby L, Meredith N. Resonance frequency analysis: Measuring implant stability and osseointegration. Compend Contin Educ Dent 1998;19:493–498,500,502; quiz 504.
16. Meredith N, Book K, Friberg B, Jemt T, Sennerby L. Resonance frequency measurements of implant stability in vivo. A cross-sectional and longitudinal study of resonance frequency measurements on implants in the edentulous and partially dentate maxilla. Clin Oral Implants Res 1997;8(3): 226–233.

chapter 3

Diagnosis and Treatment Planning

Lars G. Hollender, DDS
Michael R. Arcuri, DDS, MS
Brien R. Lang, DDS, MS

Varying degrees of functional, esthetic, and psychologic impairment can result from the loss of one tooth to the loss of the entire dentition. Fortunately, in most of these situations, dental therapy is available that can be used for the rehabilitation of those patients who experience such a loss. The placement of a dental implant with predictable success followed by prosthetic rehabilitation is a therapy that can be applied to the treatment of an edentulous space. In fact, it is an obligation on the part of the clinician to offer implant therapy to a patient as a treatment option if conditions indicate that the patient is a candidate for such treatment. The decision as to whether or not implant therapy is an option for a patient can be made by adhering to the data-gathering process outlined in Box 3-1.

The key to the success of any dental treatment is a well-organized and well-performed data-gathering process. This process is best performed when the clinician follows sequential steps in gathering information, which begin at the initial pa-

> **Box 3-1** An outline for planning implant therapy
>
> 1. The patient examination
>   - General health
>   - Dental health
>   - Radiographic evaluations
>   - Photographic record
> 2. The diagnostic mounting
> 3. Presentation of the treatment plan to the patient

tient examination. The assembled information, combined with a diagnostic mounting of dental casts made of the patient's arches, will be used to differentiate between patients who can be best served by placement of implants and those who would be better served by conventional prosthodontic therapy. If implants are selected as an appropriate treatment option for the patient, the information gathered throughout this process will also assist in the selection of the surgical protocols to be followed and define the needed prosthodontic therapy.

Patient Examination

A great deal of important information can be obtained during the initial examination about the overall demeanor and attitude of the patient. For example, the patient who presents the clinician with a bag of recently fabricated prostheses, or who wears mismatched sets of dentures at the examination appointment, may have unrealistic expectations. Patients who claim they have "special needs" and express great doubt that anyone can successfully treat them are poor candidates for implants. However, these types of patients may also turn out to be successful implant patients if additional diagnostic procedures are performed prior to implant therapy.

The patient's past medical and dental history; examination of the hard and soft tissues; and radiographic evaluations, including panoramic, cephalometric, periapical and occlusal films, and possibly tomographic or computerized tomographic (CT) scans of the jaw(s) under consideration, provide valuable diagnostic information needed for optimal treatment planning.

General health

A thorough review of the medical history is important to determine whether a patient is a candidate for dental implants. Certain medical conditions may preclude the patient from undergoing implant treatment. Any disease process that would compromise complete healing should exclude a patient from implant therapy. Diabetes, osteoporosis, and cardiac and vascular diseases might immediately come to mind as potential conditions of concern; however, these diseases, when controlled, have not been reported as contraindicating implant treatment.[1] When present, these conditions require only that conventional precautions be followed throughout surgical intervention and prosthetic care to ensure success. Neither age nor prolonged steroid medications are considered factors that would eliminate a patient from implant therapy.

Medical contraindications

Medical contraindications primarily concern the ability of the patient's tissues to heal. Implants should not be placed while a patient is undergoing treatments that cause a systemic impairment of healing, such as chemotherapy for the treatment of cancer and antimetabolic therapy (eg, methotrexate) for the treatment of arthritis. Patients who suffer from uncontrolled diabetes should also forgo implant treatment until the disease is properly managed, as should patients with seriously impaired cardiovascular function. Active addictions to drugs, including alcohol, should also be considered medical contraindications to treatment with implants.

Patients with a history of radiation therapy to the maxillomandibular region should not be considered for implant treatment under routine protocols. Implants may be successfully placed in irradiated bone, but the procedures for placement and restoration of the implants are still in the investigative phase of development.

Psychiatric contraindications

Psychiatric contraindications are often difficult to identify. These conditions may be undiagnosed or unreported by the patient. Blomberg has identified the following as psychiatric contraindications to treatment.[2]

- Psychotic syndromes, such as schizophrenia or paranoia
- Severe character disorders and neurotic syndromes, such as hysteria and borderline personality disorders
- Dysmorphophobia (an irrational fear of deformity) or extreme and unrealistic expectations and demands regarding the cosmetic results of the operation rather than the effects of retention problems
- Syndromes of cerebral lesions and presenile dementia
- Alcohol or drug abuse, if not diagnosed with great certainty as secondary to the oral problem

Patients with impaired psychologic function and personality patterns of avoidance behavior should be thoroughly examined by appropriate medical colleagues before they are accepted as implant candidates. Psychiatric disorders such as psychotic tendencies and severe neuroses are general health conditions that should cause the clinician to question implant therapy as the treatment of choice for these patients. Drug abuse and chemical dependency are habits that probably would impair patient compliance and oral hygiene motivation, which are needed for any complex reconstruction, including those involving dental implants.

Patients in reasonably good general health and who appear psychologically stable are good candidates for implants. Above all else, patients must demonstrate that they are motivated to pursue treatment and that they will cooperate with recommendations made by the treating clinician(s).

Dental health

The dental history may give some insight to the patient's previous prosthetic experiences, dental knowledge, and expectations. Pretreatment evaluations of the dental health of a patient may vary as performed by different clinicians. However, the following steps must be considered because of their importance in diagnosis and treatment planning.

- Examination of soft and hard tissues
- Imaging, including but not limited to radiographic examinations and photographs
- Diagnostic mounting

Examination of soft and hard tissues

The condition of the mucous membranes, the health of the jaws, and the status of the teeth are the primary local health factors to be considered in the soft and hard tissues examination. Healthy oral mucosa is required for implant placement, and any soft or hard tissue pathosis must be treated before implant therapy can be considered. Herpetic stomatitis, candidiasis, denture-induced stomatitis, and hyperplastic tissues are conditions that negatively influence treatment success. Tooth impactions, bone cysts, root fragments, and residual bone infections contraindicate implant therapy, and the presence of a benign bone tumor in the jaw would also eliminate a patient from implant treatment until these conditions are treated.

Every edentulous space potentially can be restored with dental implants. However, all reasonable types of prosthetic reconstructive procedures must also be considered during the examination. Implants are one option among the prosthodontic services available. The prosthetic choices are influenced by the adjacent teeth with respect to their periodontal health and the presence or absence of existing restorations. The pulp health, presence of caries, esthetic requirements, and shape, contours, and bone density of the residual ridge in the edentulous space can also affect the decision about which treatment option to suggest to the patient. The alignment and orientation of the adjacent teeth can be an influence on whether to restore the edentulous space using a conventional fixed partial denture or to restore the space using implants.

The oral examination should include measurements of any edentulous spaces.[3] A space of 7.0 mm in width between neighboring teeth is considered necessary for placement of single implants that are 3.75 or 4.0 mm in diameter. For spaces that are only 5.0 to 6.0 mm in width, narrower implants are available. If the space available is a concern and could potentially compromise therapy, then implants should not be placed.

A minimum vertical distance from the mucosa to the opposing dentition is needed for the implant prosthetic components. In some situations, the space available will be adequate for a transmucosal or abutment component followed by the placement of a conventional crown onto the abutment. Other situations may necessitate the design of an implant prosthetic crown that originates at the implant level as a single unit to accommodate the available vertical space. In situations with a greatly resorbed ridge, a greater vertical height in the edentulous space will result in the need for a very long prosthetic unit or clinical crown, which may compromise the eventual esthetic results. This diagnostic information is essential for the development of a treatment plan to be presented to the patient.

Good oral hygiene is necessary for long-term implant success, but completely or partially edentulous patients with extremely poor oral hygiene need not necessarily be excluded from implant treatment. After such patients are educated about the significance of good oral hygiene, however, it is advisable that the patient be subjected to a trial period of several months to demonstrate good oral hygiene practices. If the patient achieves and maintains adequate hygiene levels during this time period, the patient could then be considered for implant treatment.

Imaging

It is important to perform a radiographic survey during the initial patient evaluation. The initial radiographs may include but are not limited to panoramic, cephalometric, occlusal, and periapical radiographs. The quantity and quality of jawbone are two important factors to consider in patient selection for implant therapy (see Boxes 3-2 and 3-3).[4]

The preimplantation imaging aims at identification of pathologic changes in the regions intended for implants, assessment of bony structures and dimensions, and the location of important anatomic structures, such as the mandibular canal, mental foramen, and floor of the maxillary sinus. To accomplish this, a radiographic three-dimensional evaluation is needed in the majority of cases. A three-dimensional evaluation will also provide information about the buccal and lingual contours of the bone, including concavities and irregularities that may interfere with successful implant placement. In many cases, such information may result in the use of implants of different dimensions versus implants that were planned with only a two-dimensional evaluation.

Box 3-2 Assessment of bone quantity according to Lekholm and Zarb[4]

A Most of the alveolar ridge is present.
B Moderate residual ridge resorption has occurred.
C Advanced residual ridge resorption has occurred and only basal bone remains.
D Some resorption of the basal bone has taken place.
E Extreme resorption of the basal bone has taken place.

Box 3-3 Assessment of bone quality according to Lekholm and Zarb[4]

1 Almost the entire jaw is comprised of homogenous compact bone.
2 A thick layer of compact bone surrounds a core of dense trabecular bone.
3 A thin layer of cortical bone surrounds a core of dense trabecular bone of favorable strength.
4 A thin layer of cortical bone surrounds a core of low-density trabecular bone.

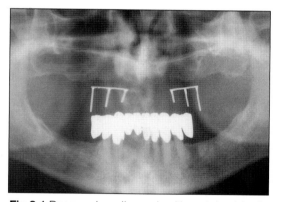

Fig 3-1 Panoramic radiograph with metal guides in the maxilla.

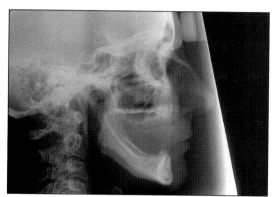

Fig 3-2 Lateral cephalometric radiograph showing the sagittal midline dimensions of the mandibular and maxillary anterior regions.

Typically, panoramic and/or intraoral radiographs are combined with tomographic images, which render cross-sectional views of the implant region. Panoramic and lateral (cephalometric) radiographs of the jaws can be used to obtain adequate three-dimensional information regarding the anterior regions of the maxilla and mandible (Figs 3-1 and 3-2). CT is frequently applied to obtain cross-sectional images of the jaws, but conventional tomography can give the desired cross-sectional information at a lower cost, and many times also at lower doses of radiation.

Irrespective of the imaging modalities applied, it is very important that the radiographic technicians and other practitioners involved in the radiologic part of the implant treatment have adequate training and understanding of the principles of successful imaging. It is particularly important to be able to identify images of suboptimal quality, through which erroneous information might be obtained about dimensions and locations of critical structures.

In all preimplantation imaging procedures, an imaging guide or stent should be used to indicate not only the location of the intended implant but also the ideal direction of the implant. Such guides must be customized to the imaging modality. Thus the guide typically used for CT, with crown replicas in acrylic containing a contrasting agent such as barium, is not as well suited for conventional tomography. This is because the image of such a crown will be superimposed on the blurred images of neighboring crowns or crown replicas. For conventional tomography, small metallic rods, or crown replicas in acrylic with a thin lead foil glued to the surface, are better suited. Also, if several implants are planned for the same area of the jaw, the guide for each individual implant site should have a unique shape or feature so that it cannot be confused with other guides if conventional tomography is used.

Panoramic radiography

The panoramic radiograph provides an enlarged image of the jaws. Usually the magnification factor is between 1.25 and 1.30 for ordinary panoramic radiographs. This magnification factor is valid only for the central parts of the layer in focus (focal trough). Outside this central part, the vertical and horizontal magnification increases in areas that are closer to the radiation source and decreases in areas that are closer to the film. The change in vertical magnification is smaller than that in the horizontal. Furthermore, the change in horizontal magnification is greater in the anterior region than in the posterior. Since many patients are not placed ideally in the panoramic machine, horizontal dimensions in the panoramic image may deviate significantly from the true dimensions. Vertical dimensions are more reliable, but apart from the influence of patient positioning, the anatomic shape of the jaws may introduce errors as a result of the projection angle (from below) of the panoramic machine and the angle or shape of the alveolar process. For instance, the vertical dimension of the alveolar process in the anterior region of the mandible may be exaggerated in the panoramic radiograph because of the angle of the symphyseal region in the sagittal plane. Similar exaggeration of the vertical dimension may occur in the posterior region of the mandible because of the projection of the lingual "shelf" of bone above the real superior border of the alveolar ridge. Also, the buccal location of the mental foramen may create an overestimation of the distance between the alveolar crest and the foramen, since the crest is usually more lingual and therefore will be projected more superiorly. On the other hand, a lingual location of the mandibular canal may lead to an impression of a shorter distance between the canal and the alveolar crest. Also, the position of the genu of the mandibular canal can be projected more anteriorly than in reality, particularly if the patient is placed forward in the panoramic machine. The panoramic radiograph also offers an image with less geometric resolution than the intraoral radiograph, which means that some of the bony trabeculation seen in the intraoral radiograph will not be apparent in the panoramic radiograph.

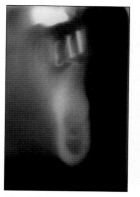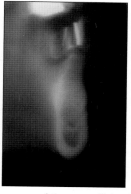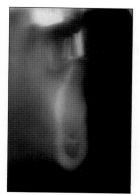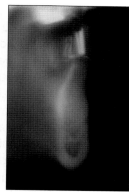

Fig 3-3 Conventional tomograms of the mandible showing the mandibular canal and mental foramen, as well as the tapering width of the superior parts of the alveolar ridge. Note the relative unsharpness of the cortical borders due to blurring of adjacent parts.

Conventional tomography

Cross-sectional images of the jaws should be obtained with the tomographic plane at right angles to the buccal and lingual plates and at a right angle to the vertical long axis of the jaw section (Fig 3-3). Deviation from this requirement will cause geometric distortion and consequently provide erroneous information about jaw dimensions and the locations of critical structures relative to the alveolar crest. It will also impair the identification of the borders of the jaw in the radiographs. Small deviations from the ideal are less important. However, significant deviations can occur in the premolar regions of the maxilla with regard to the position of the floor of the maxillary sinus, since the floor often curves upward and thus will not be imaged at a right angle. The thickness of the sharp image layer should be between 2 and 4 mm. The advantage with thinner layers is that structures not be-

longing to the layer are blurred more efficiently than when thicker layers are used. The advantage with thicker layers is that structures that may not produce enough contrast to be seen in thinner layer images will be visible in the thicker layer images. For instance, the mandibular canal may be identified unequivocally in a 4-mm-thick tomographic layer but not—or more ambiguously—in a 2- or 1-mm-thick layer.

In conventional tomography, dense structures outside the tomographic layer, such as teeth, will cause "ghost images" and may at times compromise identification of the true shape and confines of the alveolar bone. Also, a thick, dense cortical plate will produce a diffuse dense structure around the "real" image of the cortical plate, preventing the identification of the true borders of the section and causing misinterpretation of the width of the cortical plate. All tomographic images are enlarged (typically be-

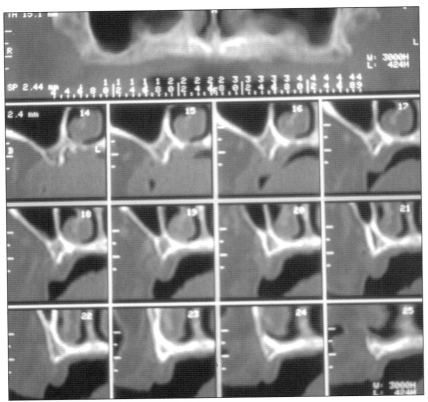

Fig 3-4 Reformatted CT images of the right maxilla.

tween 1.25 and 1.5 times), so measurements of dimensions must be adjusted to obtain actual values.

Computerized tomography

This imaging modality renders tomographic images of the jaws in practically any direction, usually with easily identifiable borders of the alveolar bone and anatomic structures such as the mandibular canal (Fig 3-4). Usually axial sections are obtained directly from a contiguous helical scanning and are used thereafter for reconstructions of desired imaging planes of the implant regions.

As with conventional tomography, these planes should be at right angles to the buccal and lingual cortical plates and at a right angle to the vertical long axis of the jaw. There are no disturbing ghost images from structures outside the imaged section in computerized tomography, but when structures with very high density such as metal objects are located within the imaged section, artifacts are produced that may render the image useless. Most CT imaging software will give actual (not distorted or enlarged) values for dimensions. Depending on the window used for the CT images, the width of the cortical bone will vary. So-called volume averaging may introduce minor errors, which are probably of little consequence for treatment planning.

Photographs

Intraoral and extraoral photographs have proven invaluable as a record of the conditions that existed before treatment began. Obviously, they are also important as a visual record during the treatment planning stages of implant therapy.

Diagnostic Mounting

Dental casts mounted on a dental articulator, along with intraoral and extraoral photographs, are essential in helping to select appropriate treatment options. The diagnostic mounting should provide the answers to several questions that must be addressed by the clinician.

1. Would the missing tooth structure or the edentulous space be better restored or replaced by a fixed or removable partial denture?
2. Does an acceptable occlusal plane exist, and if not, could one be developed in conjunction with implant treatment?
3. Is there adequate interarch space for the implant and restoration?
4. Is there adequate distance between teeth adjacent to the edentulous space for placement of an implant and restoration?

Securing dental casts of the patient and mounting these casts on the dental articulator will provide a great deal of information about the existing oral conditions that may not be obvious during the oral examination.

The diagnostic mounting offers the clinician the opportunity to design optimal occlusal contacts and to determine the need for additional restorative care.

Initial selection of the implant design for a patient can be made from the diagnostic mounting. Once the implant has been selected, the choice of surgical approach can be considered. Clearly, the mounted casts can help the members of the implant team to decide the number of implants that will be needed and the best positions for their placement in the bone.

The design of the implant prosthesis can also be initiated with the diagnostic mounting. The definitive prosthesis will obviously differ, depending on the location and dimensions of the edentulous space and the success achieved in implant placement. Single-tooth replacement, multiple-tooth spans in partially edentulous jaws, and the totally edentulous arch are the most frequent clinical situations treated with implants. The presence or absence of specific factors in each of these situations, as observed clinically and/or determined from the diagnostic mounting, is a determinant in the decision to use implants.

In general, the absence of one or more teeth may be an indication for implant therapy, provided that the patient understands the treatment, is able to maintain the prosthesis hygienically, and has no conditions that would impair the development of osseointegration.

Long-standing short edentulous spaces might be better suited for restoration with a fixed partial denture rather than implants. This condition often has bony topography with buccal concavities, which may make successful placement of an implant difficult because of limited available bone.

Irregular cusp heights in the posterior dentition may result in premature occlusal contacts and interferences during lateral jaw movements that could result in unwanted stresses being transmitted to the implants, which may decrease the long-term success of the implant.

If minimal space exists between the edentulous ridge and the opposing teeth, and the roots of adjacent teeth converge on the edentulous space, then damage could occur to the adjacent tooth root structures when implants are placed. When the coronal proximity to adjacent teeth is limited, the development of less than optimal embrasure and occlusal contours in the restoration may be a problem. Inadequate interarch space may make fabrication of the restoration difficult, producing less than optimal esthetic and functional results.

A diagnostic waxup should be performed using the mounted casts. This will provide information on the feasibility of developing a successful restoration. The diagnostic casts with the waxup may also be shown to the patient to demonstrate the type of restoration planned (fixed or removable) and areas of potential complications.

Finalizing the Treatment Plan

The final step prior to acceptance of a patient for implant treatment is to ensure that the patient understands the procedures, timing, projected outcomes, and cost. It is important that the patient comprehends the need for routine follow-up visits and possible periodic maintenance of the prosthesis.

As long-term data on implant therapy have accumulated, it has become apparent that the placement of an endosseous implant not only provides a source of retention and stability for a prosthesis but also generates some stimulation to the surrounding bone. This stimulation appears to inhibit the loss of alveolar bone that follows tooth extraction, which has been described as both chronic and irreversible and whose long-term effects produce numerous morphologic changes that adversely affect denture-bearing areas and facial esthetics. By decreasing bone loss, an implant provides a system for bone maintenance; this enhances the therapeutic value of implant treatment.

Indications for implant therapy in an edentulous alveolus could include any patient who meets the following requirements:

- Has adequate quality and quantity of bone available for implant placement
- Is healthy enough to undergo the surgical procedure
- Is able to maintain optimal levels of oral hygiene
- Is psychologically stable and understands implant therapy, its limitations, and its accompanying responsibilities

Presentation of the Treatment Plan to the Patient

Without general health contraindications to treatment and in the presence of favorable local conditions, the treatment plan and the kinds of restorations required, including implant therapy, should be presented in some detail to the patient. The numbers and kinds of prosthetic improvements planned and overall economic considerations are part of this presentation to the patient. The esthetic and functional desires of the patient must be discussed and evaluated to determine whether the patient has unrealistic expectations. A careful evaluation of the patient's willingness and ability to provide the necessary home care before, during, and after active treatment is also necessary. Decisions concerning immediate placement of an implant following extraction of a natural tooth should be discussed if the treatment plan calls for such therapy. The number and kinds of implants to be placed and the type of anchorage (ie, fixed or removable) also must be presented. Retention of an implant restoration (ie, screw-retained or cemented) needs to be discussed. Some treatment options may need to be deferred until the implants have osseointegrated and the results have been evaluated, at which time final decisions can be made on the prosthetic therapy. Whatever the situation, the patient should be informed about these many issues, all of which must be resolved before implant surgery begins.

References

1. Laney WR, Tolman DE. The Mayo Clinic experience with tissue-integrated prostheses. In: Albrektsson T, Zarb GA (eds). The Brånemark Osseointegrated Implant. Chicago: Quintessence, 1989:165–195.
2. Blomberg S. Psychological response. In: Brånemark P-I, Zarb GA, Albrektsson T (eds). Tissue-Integrated Prostheses: Osseointegration in Clinical Dentistry. Chicago: Quintessence, 1985:165.
3. Lekholm U, Jemt T. Principles for single tooth replacement. In: Albrektsson T, Zarb GA (eds). The Brånemark Osseointegrated Implant. Chicago: Quintessence, 1989:117–126.
4. Lekholm U, Zarb GA. Patient selection and preparation. In: Brånemark P-I, Zarb GA, Albrektsson T (eds). Tissue-Integrated Prostheses: Osseointegration in Clinical Dentistry. Chicago: Quintessence, 1985:199–209.

chapter 4

Surgical Stages of Osseointegration

Philip Worthington, MD, BSc

The surgical stages of osseointegration, in which implants are introduced into the jaw, are described in this chapter. These standardized surgical procedures are directly related to the basic research performed by Professor Per-Ingvar Brånemark and his coworkers in Sweden, and they derive from an understanding of wound healing in general and bone biology in particular.

For many commonly used endosseous implant systems, the surgery is performed in two stages separated in time by a few months: Stage 1 involves placement of the implants and stage 2 entails connection of the abutments. The idea behind the two-stage system was to minimize the risk of contamination from the oral cavity and to avoid the danger to the implants that might arise if the implants were subjected to premature loading. In other words, the intention was to optimize the circumstances for uneventful wound healing so that the process of osseointegration could begin and become well-established. Subsequent experience has shown that under certain circumstances, single-stage implant systems can be successful, and indeed if conditions are favorable, implants may even sustain immediate loading. A two-stage implant system can be used as a single-stage system with immediate connection of abutments. For the beginner, however, it seems prudent to absorb first the safe, predictable two-stage protocol.

The first surgical stage may be performed under local anesthesia, with or without sedation, or under general anesthesia. It involves preparation of the implant sites in the jawbone and the introduction of the implants into the bone in a way that inflicts minimal trauma on the tissues. The soft tissues are then closed, covering the implants. Antibiotic protection combined with sterile surgical technique will minimize the risk of infection. During the healing period that follows implant placement, the implants should generally be protected from transmitted pressure such as that which might come from an overlying denture. This allows the bone to heal and the osseointegration process to begin and become established; the healing bone grows up to and adheres to the layer of titanium oxides (or ceramic coating, such as hydroxyapatite) on the implant surface. In the average mandible, this period will be a minimum of 3 months long. In the maxilla it will be a minimum of 6 months' duration because of the looser texture and slower healing of the maxillary bone.

In the second stage of implant surgery, the buried implant is exposed and some form of abutment is connected to the implant. This abutment serves to attach the prosthesis, which is fabricated by the restorative dentist or prosthodontist. The precise type of abutment to be used depends on the details of the restorative plan. Many variations of abutment design are now available for differing situations.

Stage 1 Surgery: Implant Placement

The bone of the jaw is exposed by the reflection of a flap of mucoperiosteum. The position of the incision and the design of the flap will vary with differing situations and operator preference, but commonly the incision is placed in the buccolabial vestibule (so as to be remote from the implant sites themselves), and a flap is developed based on the tissue lingual to the alveolar ridge (Figs 4-1a and 4-1b). Having reflected a flap, the surgeon then identifies a suitable implant site; this is marked by a small round bur in the cortical bone. Attention is given to the spacing of multiple implant sites to ensure that they are not too close together. The next step is to drill a narrow cylindrical hole in the bone using a narrow twist drill (Fig 4-1c). In doing this, care must be taken to control the

angulation of the drill, bearing in mind the future prosthodontic needs. The narrow hole is then widened, using first a pilot drill that has a blunt tip with a wider cutting section behind it, and then using a wide twist drill to widen the hole to the required depth (Fig 4-1d). A countersink is then used to shape the occlusal end of the implant site to receive the flared neck of the implant (Fig 4-1e). All these steps are performed using drill speeds below 2,000 revolutions per minute and profuse cooling irrigation.

After the depth of the implant site is measured with a special gauge, site preparation is completed with a titanium tap, which is used to cut a thread on the walls of the cylindrical hole (Fig 4-1f). For this, a special drill rotating at no more than 15 revolutions per minute is used. This step is also performed with cooling irrigation. If the internal texture of the bone is found to be soft, the tapping step may be omitted and self-tapping implants used. If the bone is found to be unusually dense, the tap may have difficulty in cutting the thread in the bone, and the use of a slightly wider drill than usual (eg, 3.15-mm diameter instead of 3.0-mm diameter) will solve this problem.

When the implant site is thus prepared, an implant of suitable length may be threaded into it and gently screwed into place (Fig 4-1g). The aim is to place a series of implants into the edentulous jaw with near parallelism; absolute parallelism is not essential. For a close approximation to parallelism, the surgeon uses metal directional indicators that are temporarily placed into the holes. In this way the operator can judge the angulation of the next implant to be placed in sequence. As a rule, the prosthodontist will provide a drilling template for the surgeon to guide the placement of the implants, ie, their position, spacing, and angulation.

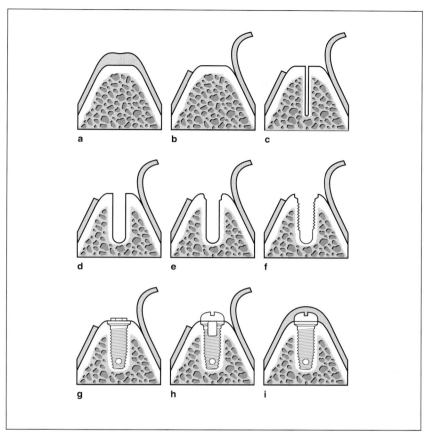

Fig 4-1 Stage 1 surgery for two-stage endosseous implant systems. The preoperative alveolar ridge appears in cross section *(a)*. The mucoperiosteal flap is raised *(b)*, and an initial hole is drilled into the bone *(c)*. This hole is then widened *(d)*, usually modified with a countersinking drill *(e)*, then threaded with a tap *(f)*. The implant is gently screwed into place *(g)*, and a cover screw is added to occlude the central space *(h)*. The mucosal flap can then be replaced to exclude the implant from the oral cavity during the healing period *(i)*.

When all the implants have been placed in the bone, the final step is to put a cover screw in the top of each implant (Fig 4-1h) so as to occlude its internal thread and to prevent connective tissue and bone from growing over and obscuring the occlusal end of the implant.

The mucoperiosteal flap is then replaced and sutured in position (Fig 4-1i). The patient should not wear a denture over the operating site for about 2 weeks. At the end of that time, the denture may be modified by the prosthodontist: The flanges may be reduced slightly, the fitting surface may be relieved over the implant sites, and the whole fitting surface may be coated with a soft lining material. The patient can then wear the modified denture during the few months of the healing period.

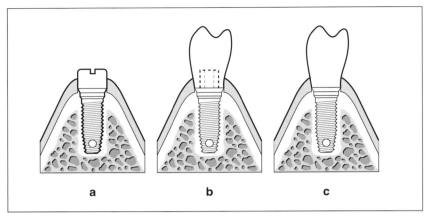

Fig 4-2 Stage 2 surgery for two-stage endosseous implant systems. The cover screws are located, removed, and replaced by an abutment cylinder that penetrates the mucosa into the mouth. A healing cap is placed first over the coronal end of the abutment cylinder (a). This is later replaced by the prosthetic component (b), which is fixed using a screw or cement (c).

Stage 2 Surgery: Abutment Connection

First, the buried implants are located by palpation and, if necessary, by probing. Under local anesthesia they are then exposed by means of a mucoperiosteal incision and, if necessary, by using a circular punch to remove overlying mucoperiosteum. This exposure allows the surgeon to remove the cover screws and to make sure that the coronal end of each implant is clean and free of overlying wisps of connective tissue and bone. The depth of the mucoperiosteum must be measured, and an abutment of suitable type and size is attached to the implant using an abutment screw and a small screwdriver, with a special clamp holding the abutment to prevent the transfer of torque to the implant itself. At this stage, the abutment will protrude into the mouth and the surrounding gingiva will be replaced and sutured into position. When all the abutment cylinders

have been placed, healing caps are attached to their coronal ends (Fig 4-2a) to allow a periodontal pack to be placed and retained under the projecting edges of the healing caps. This protects the gingiva and holds the soft tissue against the bone. Accurate seating of the abutments onto the ends of the implants is checked visually in the mouth and via radiographs. This is the first time that a radiograph is taken after implant placement.

After 1 to 2 weeks, the pack and the sutures are removed, and the patient is ready to begin the restorative phase of treatment, which involves attaching the prosthodontic components (Figs 4-2b and 4-2c).

Surgical Considerations

Maintenance of asepsis and sterility is crucial during these surgical stages. All implant surgery should be performed with due regard for standard sterile operating tech-

---

Box 4-1 Keys to implant surgery success

1. Minimize the risk of infection by:
   - Careful preparation and draping of the patient
   - Use of sterile technique under operation room conditions
   - Use of presterilized packaged components
   - Prescription of antibiotic cover

2. Minimize tissue injury with:
   - Gentle surgical technique
   - Sharp, disposable drills of increasing sizes
   - Light and intermittent drilling pressure
   - Controlled rotational drill speeds and controlled torque
   - Copious cooling irrigation

3. Avoid contamination of implant surfaces by:
   - Separation of titanium and stainless steel components and instruments
   - Use of only titanium instruments in contact with titanium components
   - Maintenance of sterile technique
   - Avoidance of contact of gloves, suction tubing, or anything other than titanium with titanium implants

---

nique and with antibiotic cover. Special care should be taken to avoid contamination of the integrating surfaces of the titanium components. The handling of the tissues should be as gentle as possible, and copious coolant should be used during all heat-generating steps. The removal of the bone should be incremental so as to minimize bony trauma and heat generation. The drills should be sharp, and the drilling pressure should be light and intermittent.

The incision for implant placement is commonly made in the labial vestibule, away from the crest of the ridge, and a flap developed that is lingually or palatally based, so that the suture line is not located directly over the implant sites. This is thought to minimize the risk of contamination of the implants from the oral cavity. In certain circumstances, a crestal incision may be preferred; for example, where the normal

vascularity of the soft tissues has been impaired by previous surgery.

When the implant system is of the single-stage (nonsubmerged) type, the implant penetrates the mucosa immediately. In such cases it is considered wiser to avoid loading the implants until after a suitable healing period. The ITI System (Straumann USA, Waltham, MA) follows this pattern.

When implants are cylindrical without threads, the thread-tapping step is omitted from site preparation. This type of implant relies on "press-fit" friction for placement into the site.

Regardless of which type of endosseous implant is used, the chances of successful osseointegration will be enhanced by adherence to certain points of surgical protocol designed to minimize tissue trauma, avoid contamination, maintain sterility, and maximize precision (Box 4-1).

chapter 5

Intraoral Implant Applications

Michael E. Razzoog, DDS, MS, MPH
Jeffrey E. Rubenstein, DMD, MS

The limited long-term success of dental implant treatment prior to the introduction of osseointegrated implants left most dentists skeptical about the routine clinical application for replacing missing teeth with implants. Most implants were unpredictable and eventually failed, with some failing more rapidly than others. Over the last 20+ years, skepticism has been replaced by renewed interest among specialists and general dentists as a result of the efforts of Per-Ingvar Brånemark and his coworkers in Sweden, who were largely responsible for introducing the concept of osseointegration.[1] In the mid-1960s, Brånemark demonstrated that implants could survive with certainty in the oral environment as long as specific biologic principles were not violated. When the principles of osseointegration are followed, the anchorage of a nonbiologic titanium implant to bone with a direct structural and functional connection between living bone and the surface of a load-carrying implant will occur. Reports in the dental literature repeatedly indicate sur-

vival rates of 95% and 85%, respectively, for the mandible and maxilla.[2] Several longitudinal studies of implants placed in edentulous jaws have been conducted to validate osseointegration, and the method has withstood this scientific scrutiny.[3–5]

Osseointegration is now considered by the dental profession as mainstream treatment for replacement of single teeth, multiple teeth, or completely missing dentitions. Reports suggest that dental implant treatment will play an ever-increasing role in oral rehabilitation well into the 21st century.

A wide array of treatment applications using implants is just beginning to be realized by oral health care providers. Dental implants have been used primarily as replacements for tooth roots or tooth-root analogs (Fig 5-1). However, implants are not limited to replacement of missing teeth. Implants have also been used with equal success for anchorage to facilitate orthodontic tooth movement, retention of facial prostheses, and prosthetic joint and limb replacements (see chapter 11). Various bone

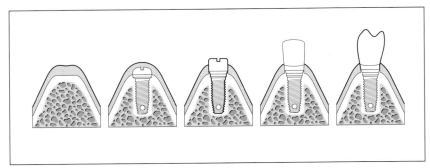

Fig 5-1 Basic process of single-tooth replacement using an endosseous screw-type implant. *(left to right)* The preoperative ridge, initial implant placement with cover screw, healing abutment placement, definitive abutment placement, final cemented crown restoration. See chapter 7 for further details on specific implant and abutment designs.

grafting techniques have been developed to facilitate the use of dental implants where such treatment was otherwise deemed impossible. An entirely new approach to develop sites for implant placement has been formulated using implants, various types of membranes, and bone grafting materials, a technique known as *guided tissue regeneration*. Clinicians have also begun to place implants immediately at the time of tooth extraction, rather than waiting months for the socket to heal. Prospective patients, otherwise dissuaded by the longer conventional treatment protocol, are seeking this more rapid approach to tooth replacement.

Information specifically relevant to potential clinical applications of dental implant treatment was revealed in the 1985–1986 National Institute for Dental Research survey of tooth loss and estimated prosthetic treatment needs in employed adults and seniors in the United States.[6] These data showed that in 1986, only 10% of 65- to 69-year-olds, 26% of 55- to 64-year-olds, 32% of 45- to 54-year-olds, and 50% of 35- to 44-year-olds did not require pros-

thodontic treatment. Most of the US population older than 35 years demonstrated patterns of tooth loss that suggested a potential for tooth replacement with dental implants.

A conservative estimate suggests a 38% increase in the need for prosthodontic services today when compared with the need cited 25 years ago. The projected unmet need for prosthodontic treatment in the year 2020 suggests a trend for increasing clinical indications for dental implant services for the future.

In 1991, there were 31 million people older than 65 years in the United States. Chester Douglass has reported that although this number will increase to 52 million by 2020, the total edentulous population will only rise from the 1991 figure of 33.6 million to 37.9 million in 2020.[7] However, the decrease in the total edentulism percentage for the entire population will be more than offset by the 79% growth in the population aged 55 years and older. The number of patients in this age category who will be partially edentulous should increase substantially.

Currently, it is estimated that 41% of people older than 40 have one or more missing teeth. Given the increase in the size of the population in need of prosthodontic services, the clinical applications for implants for single teeth and treatment of partial edentulism have the potential to grow proportionately over the next few decades.

Clinical Applications

The range of intraoral clinical applications involving dental implants is expanding. Innovative clinicians continue to explore new treatment protocols for dental implants that expand their current uses to provide comfortable, functional, and esthetically pleasing solutions for individuals with missing teeth. There is also an increasing use of implants as an alternative to conventional prosthodontic procedures, eg, replacement of a missing single tooth with an implant instead of a fixed partial denture.

The intraoral clinical applications of implants in today's dental practice include the following:

1. Treatment of the totally edentulous maxilla and mandible
2. Restoration of anterior and posterior edentulous spaces, which may or may not be bounded by natural teeth
3. Replacement of the single missing tooth
4. Provision of anchorage for orthodontic tooth movement

Totally edentulous arch

The pioneering work in osseointegration highlighted implants as a preprosthetic sur-

gical procedure used to aid totally edentulous patients who have lost not only teeth but also excessive amounts of their residual ridges as a result of bone resorption (reduction of the volume and dimensions of the maxillary and/or mandibular arch). These patients usually present with dentures that are no longer stable and retentive. Full-arch implant rehabilitation continues to be used in both the maxilla and mandible. Prospective and retrospective studies have clearly demonstrated the predictability and versatility of osseointegration in large numbers of edentulous patients who otherwise were functionally compromised or incapacitated in regard to their oral function with conventional complete dentures.[3–5] For those patients unable to function with a mandibular complete denture, an implant-retained overdenture is now considered by many as the standard of care.[8]

Surgical placement of implants into the anterior segment of the edentulous arch has provided a method of support and retention for implant overdentures where bone loss has compromised denture-bearing areas. The number of implants used is dictated by bone quality and quantity. Two or more implants used with a variety of available attachments or a splinted bar system can assist denture retention and provide an improved quality of life for the patient (Fig 5-2). Many patients seek to have the palate left uncovered when maxillary implants are used in conjunction with an implant overdenture approach. It is worth noting, however, that the palate serves as an additional base of support to assist implants with occlusal loading. Therefore, through the elimination of palatal coverage, the load distribution is borne entirely by the bone-implant interface. This may be, in part, an explanation for the higher failure rate of max-

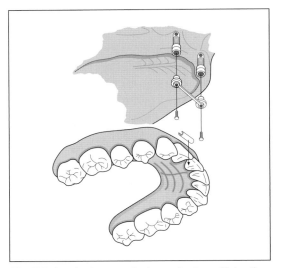

Fig 5-2 Implant-supported overdenture. Retention is provided by the bar placed between two or more implants and the posterior residual alveolar ridge.

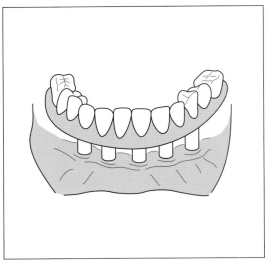

Fig 5-3 Implant-supported fixed prosthesis placed in a totally edentulous mandible.

illary implants associated with implant overdenture treatment.

Strategic placement of five or six dental implants has been shown to be very successful in providing totally edentulous patients with a full-arch, implant-supported fixed prosthesis (Fig 5-3) or an overdenture retained by splinted implant frameworks. Full-arch implant rehabilitation in both the maxilla and mandible with an appropriate selection of abutments and prosthetic designs has contributed significantly to the improved comfort, function, and appearance of thousands of patients. The combination of implants and a fixed prosthesis in the mandibular arch with a maxillary complete denture has been shown to restore oral function nearly to that of patients with an intact natural dentition.

Partially edentulous arch

Spaces previously occupied by more than one tooth

Dental implants may be used to restore partially edentulous spaces previously occupied by more than one natural tooth (Fig 5-4). The type and placement of implant(s) for support of the prosthesis varies with each patient. For example, in the case of a missing maxillary central and lateral incisor, the implant prosthesis can be either splinted, left as two independent single-tooth implant restorations, or structured as a pontic cantilevered off one implant. In other situations, the edentulous space may consist of more than two missing teeth and be lacking a posterior natural tooth abutment. There is often no conventional fixed

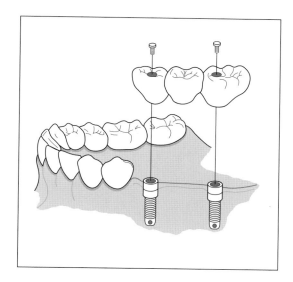

Fig 5-4 Implant-supported restoration in a partially edentulous mandible. This prosthesis is not usually attached to the adjoining natural tooth.

treatment and only a difficult removable prosthodontic treatment possible in this clinical situation.

The esthetic requirements associated with implant placement in the maxillary anterior segment ("the esthetic zone") present the greatest challenge for implant therapy. It is no longer acceptable to merely replace missing teeth in the maxillary anterior sextant. The restorative dentist and surgeon must work collaboratively to address the soft tissue architecture in such a way that the completed treatment is virtually undetectable to the discerning eye in regard to which teeth are the replacements and which are natural.

Fortunately, technical advancements and new treatment protocols have evolved for tooth replacement with dental implants. Many of the improvements have been in surgical techniques, eg, hard and soft tissue grafting, use of membranes to guide and protect grafted sites, and immediate placement of implants (in hopes of preserving bony architecture). In addition, improvements have been made in implant designs, materials, and components. These improvements include new materials such as aluminum oxide and zirconia for abutments, which aid the technician in creating a more natural appearance of the restoration, especially when the free marginal gingiva is thin and scalloped. In addition, every implant system offers abutments that can be customized by the laboratory technician or dentist to assist in creating optimal emergence profiles for the restoration.

The partially edentulous situation most frequently encountered is that of the patient with missing posterior dentition in one or both posterior sextants. These situations are also difficult to treat because of the limitations caused by anatomic structures, namely, the maxillary sinus and the inferior

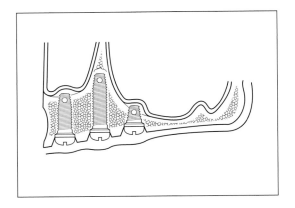

Fig 5-5 The amount of bone inferior to the maxillary sinus severely limits the potential for implant placement without additional surgical procedures. Note the difference in implant length from the anterior to the posterior maxilla.

alveolar nerve. A severely resorbed alveolar ridge or a large maxillary sinus may preclude the placement of implants in the posterior maxilla. For some patients, the canine area is sufficiently developed, and an implant placed there as well as in the first or second premolar area can provide an adequate base of abutment support, obviating the need for sinus grafting and placement of additional implants. The height of the alveolus below the floor of the sinus distal to the canine is usually less than 10 mm (Fig 5-5), which limits the number and length of implants that can be placed in that site. The most posterior part of the maxillary arch, the tuberosity, usually has a sufficient quantity of bone, but this bone is too spongy to provide predictable osseointegration. However, the dense mass of bone formed by the pterygoid process and the vertical part of the palatine bone distal to the tuberosity can sometimes provide better osseous support for implant placement. The volume of bone in the pterygomaxillary region has been found sufficient for implant placement in 80% of patients considering maxillary implant treatment.[9]

In the mandible, the walls of the mandibular canal are usually clearly visible on radiographs, and it is not uncommon that both the volume and the density of bone above the mandibular canal are sufficient to provide anchorage for a 7-, 10-, or even a 13-mm-long implant (Fig 5-6). The difficulty in placing implants in these posterior areas is that of access, which can limit placement of implants of adequate length. From the prosthodontic point of view, implants should not be placed distal to the second molar. When the height of the residual ridge above the canal is inadequate, there still may be enough bone lingual to the mandibular nerve for implant placement.

Two or more implants are normally used to restore a group of multiple missing teeth. Joining natural teeth to an implant prosthesis may be an alternative; however, the clinical situation may preclude this treatment option. There have been questions as to the difference in mobility between natural teeth and osseointegrated implants, which may result in a loss of cementation between the implant prosthesis and the adjoining natural teeth. There are clinicians and researchers

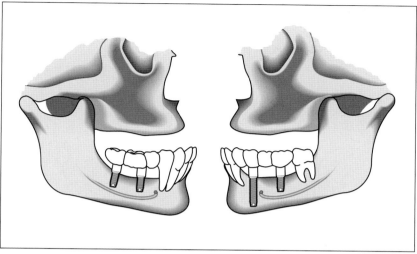

Fig 5-6 Placement of implants with respect to the mandibular canal. It is advisable to leave at least 1 mm of bone between the apex of the implant and the neurovascular bundle to prevent nerve damage.

who consider placing a crown on a natural tooth when it is joined to an implant as part of the cantilever structure of the prosthesis, rather than as part of its load-bearing abutment support. It is currently recommended that, when possible, all implant reconstructions should be freestanding on dental implants and independent of natural tooth abutment support.

In a multiple-tooth implant prosthesis, a framework is fabricated to join the prosthesis to the implant abutments. The framework may be either a cast alloy or machined titanium and be either screw- or cement-retained. During the framework fabrication, various implant components are incorporated into the prosthesis framework; the type and configuration of these components depend on the prosthesis design and type of retention/fixation.

Patients in whom the loss of the bony ridge has created anatomic defects that adversely affect the potential for a successful result have benefited from bone grafting and/or guided tissue regeneration procedures. These augmentation procedures have been used in conjunction with implants, whether placed immediately or after maturation of the grafted sites. These procedures can restore optimum ridge contours, creating a more favorable base of support for implant placement and ultimately the completed prosthesis.

Single-tooth replacement

Dental implants have been used to restore missing single teeth in situations where the use of natural tooth abutments adjacent to the edentulous space in conventional fixed prosthodontics is contraindicated (Fig 5-7).

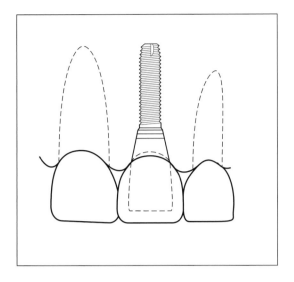

Fig 5-7 Single-tooth edentulous space restored with an implant.

A single-tooth implant restoration eliminates the need to prepare the natural teeth adjacent to the edentulous space. The use of a dental implant for a single-tooth restoration is especially advantageous in situations in which the rotation and axial alignment of potential natural tooth abutments for a fixed partial denture would result in excessive hard tissue reduction and might necessitate endodontic or orthodontic therapy as part of the treatment plan.

Esthetic and biologic demands of size and contour of the replacement restoration are important factors, and there are single-implant abutments designed to satisfy many different treatment requirements. Other important factors considered in the design of abutments for anterior single-tooth replacements are the emergence angle and profile. Even the material used for the abutment can affect the esthetic result. In the anterior maxilla, clinicians now have the choice of metal or ceramic abutments,

depending upon the esthetic requirements of the restoration. Implant abutments are available that allow for the creation of a crown that can be united with the implant abutment by either a retention screw or with cement.

Implants as anchorage for orthodontic tooth movement

Orthodontic tooth movement has always been limited to action-reaction reciprocal force mechanics. Extraoral headgear to facilitate retraction of maxillary molars is currently the most effective way of obtaining anchorage for orthodontic movement. Implants have been placed in the posterior mandible and used to retract the entire dentition in both the maxilla and mandible.[10] Implants have been used effectively for retraction and correction of a Class III anterior crossbite malocclusion in patients with missing molar teeth. The use of implants for orthodontic anchorage has been shown to be an effective adjunctive tool to facilitate orthodontic treatment, especially when natural teeth are missing in areas where anchorage is required. Implant abutments are able to support forces ranging from 150 to 400 g during the clinical course of orthodontic treatment.[10] The use of implants permits unidirectional tooth movement without reciprocal action. An implant may thus be used in place of a molar tooth (or teeth) to act as an abutment that can facilitate orthodontic treatment. Whenever implants are used as part of orthodontic treatment, the restorative dentist must be part of the treatment planning before the implants are placed. In most circumstances, the patient expects that the implant(s) will eventually be incorporated into the final prosthesis. The integration of implants into a treatment plan that includes their use as orthodontic anchorage demands close cooperation between the orthodontist, implant surgeon, and restorative dentist.

Technical Advances and New Protocols for Intraoral Applications

Immediate implant placement

The placement of an implant into an extraction site immediately after the removal of periodontally involved teeth is currently being advocated by some clinicians as an alternative to waiting 6 to 12 months for bone healing to occur before placing an implant.[11] If enough bone exists below the tooth apex, then endosseous implants can be placed at the time of extraction. Although a higher failure rate for the immedi-

ate placement of implants has been observed, limited clinical reports appear to suggest that this approach is reasonably safe and effective.

The advantages of immediate implant placement include decreased time from extraction to completion of the final prosthesis, fewer surgical procedures, and a greater likelihood that some patients will consider and accept implant treatment. A potentially greater risk of infection is the most significant concern versus the more conventional delayed implant placement approach. There are inherently more bacteria present in a mouth with periodontally involved teeth than in a completely edentulous mouth, and contamination of the surgical site during immediate implant placement is a distinct possibility.[12] More clinical studies are needed to validate the benefits of immediate implant placement and to determine the mechanisms of failure.

Guided tissue regeneration

A factor of extreme importance in the clinical application of implants in the anterior region of the mouth is lack of bone volume. To generate bone for implant placement sites deemed to be deficient, guided tissue regeneration has been suggested as an adjunctive treatment. This procedure is based on the regeneration of periodontal structures using progenitor cells, which have the potential to form cementum, the periodontal ligament, and alveolar bone, to reconfigure a bony defect into a site with more ideal anatomy. Epithelial/mucosal cells that are not capable of rebuilding periodontal tissues are of necessity excluded from contaminating and interfering with the healing wound. Physical barriers in the form of membranes are used to prevent migration of epithelial cells and cells originating from the connective tissue into the wound. According to this principle, a selective osteogenesis can be stimulated to fix defective bone architecture, thereby making implant placement possible.

The guidance of cell ingrowth originating from bone is accomplished by isolating the defect from the adjacent epithelial tissues with a membrane having a pore size that will not allow the penetration of epithelial cells. Additionally, a space is created into which progenitor cells capable of inducing bone formation can migrate, proliferate, and differentiate into osteoblasts and osteocytes. When the space between the membrane and the implant is stabilized with new bone growth, the membrane is removed. With this membrane technique, complete regeneration of bone defects around implants has been achieved.[13–15] Further research to expand the potential of guided tissue regeneration is needed.

Connection of Prostheses to Implants

Major advancements in the implant abutment design for the implant prosthesis have recently taken place. Innovations in both the materials used to fabricate abutments and the means by which a prosthesis is connected to the abutment(s) (ie, screw versus cement retention) mean that a variety of treatment options to restore dental implants are available.

Abutment materials

Abutments are fabricated from either metal or ceramic materials, depending upon the esthetic and functional requirements of the individual patient's treatment. Metal abutments can be provided by the implant manufacturer as machined titanium components, waxed to specified contours, and cast by the dental laboratory in a gold alloy, or they can be computer-designed and/or machined (CAD/CAM). In the anterior portions of the dental arch, especially the maxilla, ceramic abutments have more recently gained popularity. Ceramic abutments (Fig 5-8) are fabricated by manufacturers in either aluminum oxide or zirconia and are fabricated by a CAD/CAM approach, from a wax pattern, or using rotary instruments. Proponents of the use of ceramic abutments in the anterior maxilla, the "esthetic zone," point to the tooth color of the abutment below the gingival margin as an advantage in achieving a more natural-appearing restoration, in contrast to the gray shadow that is sometimes evident with a metal abutment. Ceramic abutments are especially indicated for patients with thin mucosa and high lip lines where excessive gingival display is evident. These nonmetallic abutments, while fabricated of strong materials comparable to titanium or cast metal abutments, might be more likely to fracture under heavy occlusal loads. As in all aspects of dental care there often is a trade-off between functional and esthetic requirements for any restoration. It is essential to clearly inform the patient about the risks and benefits of treatment options regarding choice of materials.

Connection of abutments to prostheses

Early designs of implant prostheses were screw retained. This meant that each abutment was fixed to the dental implant with

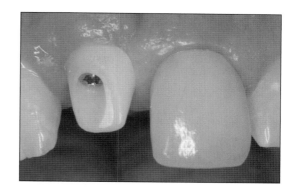

Fig 5-8 Custom ceramic abutment prior to cementation of the final crown restoration.

an abutment screw, and the prosthesis was then screwed to each abutment with a prosthetic retaining screw. The screw access channel was then covered with some form of restorative material, which could be removed if necessary to provide access to the prosthetic retaining screws, thus making the prosthesis easily retrievable. The screw-retained design has served and continues to serve many patients. However, some practitioners have questioned whether this method is appropriate for all implant prosthesis designs. It was felt by some that the screw access channel created an esthetic compromise. Other clinicians believed screw access holes compromised their ability to develop and maintain optimal occlusal contacts.

Dental laboratories throughout the United States confirm that currently the majority of implant-retained restorations are now designed to be cemented to some form of a customized abutment. An abutment can be custom-designed and fabricated in two ways: (1) The dentist can modify the abutment in the patient's mouth, making an impression and treating the abutment in a manner similar to that of a natural tooth preparation, or (2) the dentist can make an impression of the implant position, creating a cast on which the laboratory technician fabricates an abutment. Either approach results in the creation of custom abutments that are used for cemented implant restorations.

Summary

The restorative options for implant prostheses have evolved and will continue to evolve. The field has rapidly expanded, with a wide array of options now available. The uninitiated clinician's task is to become knowledgeable about, as well as familiar and comfortable with, the restorative options so that appropriate diagnosis and treatment planning and successful treatment can be accomplished.

References

1. Brånemark P-I. Introduction to osseointegration. In: Brånemark P-I, Zarb GA, Albrektsson T (eds). Tissue-Integrated Prostheses: Osseointegration in Clinical Dentistry. Chicago: Quintessence, 1985: 11–77.

2. Schnitman PA, Shulman LB. Recommendations on the Consensus Development Conference on Dental Implants. J Am Dent Assoc 1979;98:373.

3. Adell R, Eriksson B, Lekholm U, Brånemark P-I, Jemt T. A long-term follow-up study of osseointegrated implants in the treatment of totally edentulous jaws. Int J Oral Maxillofac Implants 1990; 5:347–359.

4. Adell R, Lekholm U, Rockler B, Brånemark P-I. A 15-year study of osseointegrated implants in the treatment of the edentulous jaw. Int J Oral Surg 1981;10:387–416.

5. Albrektsson T, Bergman B, Folmer T, et al. A multi-center report of osseointegrated oral implants. J Prosthet Dent 1988;60:75–84.

6. Meskin LH, Brown LJ, Brunell JA, Warren GB. Patterns of tooth loss and accumulated prosthetic treatment potential in U.S. employed adults and seniors 1985–86. Gerodontics 1988;4:126–135.

7. Douglass CW, Shih A, Ostry L. Will there be a need for complete dentures in the United States in 2020? J Prosthet Dent 2002;87:5–8.

8. The McGill Consensus Statement on Overdentures. Int J Prosthodont 2002;15:413–414.

9. Tulasne J-F. Implant treatment of missing posterior dentition. In: Laney WR, Tolman DE (eds). Tissue Integration in Oral, Orthopedic, and Maxillofacial Reconstruction. Chicago: Quintessence, 1992:103–105.

10. Higuchi K, Slack JM. The use of titanium fixtures for intraoral anchorage to facilitate orthodontic tooth movement. In: Laney WR, Tolman DE (eds). Tissue Integration in Oral, Orthopedic, and Maxillofacial Reconstruction. Chicago: Quintessence, 1992:303–307.

11. Krump JL, Barnett BG. The immediate implant: A treatment alternative. Int J Oral Maxillofac Implants 1991;6:19–23.

12. Dzink JL, Tanner ACR, Haffajee AD, Socransky SS. Gram-negative species associated with active destructive periodontal lesions. J Clin Periodontol 1985;12:648–659.

13. Wachtel HC, Langford A. Guided bone regeneration next to osseointegrated implants in humans. Int J Oral Maxillofac Implants 1991;6: 127–135.

14. Dahlin C, Sennerby L, Lekholm U, Linde A, Nyman S. Generation of new bone around titanium implants using a membrane technique: An experimental study in rabbits. Int J Oral Maxillofac Implants 1989;4:19–25.

15. Dahlin C, Gottlow J, Linde A, Nyman S. Healing of bone defects by guided tissue regeneration. Plast Reconstr Surg 1988;81:672–676.

chapter 6

Biomechanics

John B. Brunski, MS, PhD

This chapter provides basic biomechanical principles for treatment planning with dental implants. While these principles will go a long way toward ensuring a satisfactory treatment outcome, they cannot guarantee success. The reason for stopping short of a guarantee is that implant dentistry has not yet reached the stage where a completely documented "building code" exists for implant treatment. Implant dentistry is still a relatively young discipline, with new implant systems, new abutment systems, and new research on bone biology emerging monthly. Moreover, even with our best current biomechanical models for prediction of load distributions among multiple implants supporting a prosthesis, none of these models has been thoroughly tested and verified against actual in vivo data from patients. Hence, there is considerably more to be done to better understand implant biomechanics and the full implications of implant loading in relation to bone biology at the bone-implant interface. However, once these unresolved issues have been thoroughly addressed, the field will move from an era of "enlightened empiricism" into a time when clinicians will have the ability to guide patients about expected treatment outcomes based on evidence-based biomechanical analyses.

This chapter outlines some analytic tools and approaches that can assist a clinician in organizing a treatment plan for implant rehabilitation. Encyclopedic references to the in-depth literature are not provided, since this is available in some recent reviews.[1-3] A review of definitions of the term *osseointegration* is presented, emphasizing that biomechanics is embedded in the origin of that term. Key mechanical terms are then defined, including forces and moments (torques), which are essential in developing a better understanding of the biomechanics of implant therapy. Biting forces on prostheses are discussed, as well as attempts to solve the main problem of interest: How does one predict the distribution of forces and moments on implants that support prostheses? In answering this question, the chapter reviews models for predicting these loads and identifies key factors that affect the distribution of forces and moments among implants, including the stiffness of implants in bone, the properties of the prosthesis, and the nature of the abutment-prosthesis connection. Unfortunately, in-depth discussion of additional important topics such as stress and strain, material failure, stress transfer at the bone-implant interface, and interrelationships between bone biology and mechanical loading are beyond the scope of this introductory text; however, again, recent publications may be consulted, should the reader desire more detailed information.[1,2]

Definition of Osseointegration

Osseointegration has been defined in a number of ways depending on the vantage point and the scale of interest, but in all cases there is an implicit biomechanical meaning of the term. Consider the following meanings taken from a recent textbook. First, from the clinical, macroscopic view, an oral implant may be called osseointegrated if "it provides a stable and apparently immobile support of a prosthesis under functional loads without pain, inflammation or loosening."[4] Second, from a more mechanical view, an implant is called osseointegrated if "there is no progressive relative motion between the implant and surrounding living bone and marrow under functional levels and types of loading for the entire life of the patient."[4] Third, from the microscopic, biophysical point of view, note how the following description focuses on

the mechanical bone-implant contact at the osseointegrated interface:

Osseointegration implies that, at the light microscopic and electron microscopic levels, the identifiable components of tissue within a thin zone of an [implant] surface are identified as normal bone and marrow constituents that continuously grade into normal bone structure surrounding the fixture [implant]. This implies that mineralized tissue is found to be in contact with the [implant] over most of the surface within nanometers [1 nm = 10^{-9} m] so that no functionally significant intervening material exists at the interface.[4]

Beyond these definitions, the most significant point is that the literature has established that implant fixation via osseointegration allows highly predictable, long-term functional clinical performance of implant-supported prostheses in both fully and partially edentulous patients. In this context, it is interesting to note that biomechanics also plays a major role in explaining why problems sometimes develop at the osseointegrated interface, as in (1) failure to develop integration in the first place or (2) failure of an already established osseointegrated interface after loading has begun.

For example, it is known that implants can sometimes fail to become osseointegrated in the first place, and that typically this happens if the clinical conditions of implant use permit excessive relative motion (also called *micromotion*) at the bone-implant interface during the early healing period. A more detailed discussion of relative motion appears elsewhere,[1,5–8] but the basic idea is that relative motion occurs when an implant is not firmly fixed within the surgical site and is therefore able to move relative to the bony site when the implant is loaded either directly or indirectly. The consequence of such early postoperative implant "looseness" in the wounded surgical site is that—for reasons yet to be fully identified—the interface does not heal via bone regeneration; instead, it repairs itself with nonmineralized fibrous tissue encapsulation, which is not as predictable as osseointegration for implant function in the long term. Interestingly, there is evidence that formation of fibrous tissue in cases of micromotion is largely independent of the biomaterial used for the implant.[8] However, at present, we do not fully understand either (1) the exact type and amount of micromotion that leads to the formation of such nonosseous tissue or (2) the cell and molecular mechanisms underlying such tissue formation. These are topics of current research,[7] especially given the increased interest in immediate loading of implants, which carries with it the risk of implant micromotion.

There is a second way that biomechanics is central to problems with implants: Starting from a properly healed, osseointegrated state, which for purposes of this discussion we can define as undisturbed bone regeneration having occurred around the implant, osseointegration can be lost if the implant is subsequently "overloaded." That is, if there are excessively large forces and/or moments on the implant, it has been observed that there can be a progressive loss of interfacial bone-implant contact (typically starting at the crestal region), which can worsen over a period of weeks to months if the excessive loading conditions continue unabated.[9–11] Eventually, the implant and/or interfacial bone fails and the implant can no longer function as a fixed

support for a prosthesis. As in the case of relative motion, the cellular and molecular details underlying failure by overload have yet to be fully determined. But the evidence strongly supports the idea that for both failure by relative motion and failure by overload, biomechanics is intimately involved in the mechanisms. Indeed, biomechanics is critical to the success and failure of oral implants and should therefore be a part of the academic background of any clinician wanting to treat patients appropriately with implants.

Relevance of Biomechanics in Case Planning

Another obvious way to appreciate the relevance of biomechanics comes from consideration of a typical problem that can arise during case planning. For example, suppose a clinician wants to place oral implants in the mandible or maxilla so that a certain type of full-arch prosthesis will be supported. An initial question is: How many implants should be placed, and how should they be spaced and oriented over the length of the arch to ensure the best results? Should the implants be spaced out as widely as possible over the available distance, or is it just as effective to place them close to one another? Does it matter if some implants are tilted? Is there any problem if some of the implants are placed in very dense bone, while others are placed in somewhat "softer" cancellous bone? Even more confounding: Do the answers to the previous questions change for immediate as opposed to delayed loading?

While our current knowledge base makes it difficult to answer the above questions,

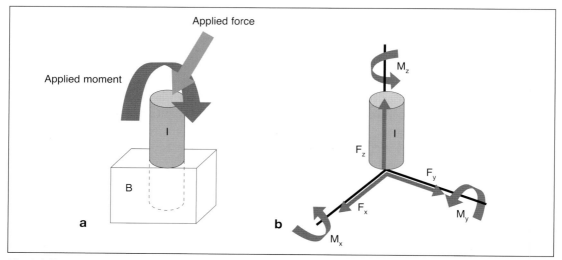

Fig 6-1 Force and moment components resisted by an idealized fixed support. *(a)* A loaded implant (I) supported by bone (B). The implant is meant to act as a fixed support. *(b)* Reactions at a fixed support. The bone-implant interface exerts forces (F) and moments (M) on the implant. (Adapted from Hibbeler[12] with permission from Pearson Education.)

they can be boiled down to the following three basic questions that arise in almost all implant therapies:

1. What are the forces and moments exerted on the prosthesis and implants supporting the prosthesis?
2. As we plan a case, or even after the prosthesis is inserted and we are interested in its performance, how can we predict the load distribution among the one or more implants that support the prosthesis, and what factors influence the load distribution?
3. What are safe versus dangerous loads on implants and surrounding bone?

A good understanding of current answers to these questions can help prevent failure of any part of the implant case, including the prosthesis, supporting implants, and supporting biologic tissues. As noted before, this chapter is limited mainly to the first two questions; other literature can be consulted for information on the third, which is a more complicated topic.

Loading of Prostheses and Implants

In elementary mechanics, the purpose of any oral or craniofacial implant is to act as a fixed support (Fig 6-1). In common experience, a good example of a fixed support is a common household nail or screw driven into a piece of wood; the nail or screw is anchored in such a way that it can resist forces and twisting actions (moments) applied to it in all directions. Ideally, an oral implant should also be able to function in vivo as a fixed support. Moreover, the implant ought to be anchored strongly enough in bone so that neither the implant nor the surrounding interfacial bone fails under the expected loading. Here the importance of studying forces and moments becomes obvious.

Forces

During mastication, the masticatory muscles act to move the jaws, causing the teeth to shred and crush food into particles. During mastication, a number of factors determine the forces on the prosthesis and any teeth or implants that support the prosthesis. To discuss these factors using accurate language, it is appropriate to introduce basic concepts of mechanics, including the definitions of *force* and *force components*. (*Moment* and *moment components* will be discussed shortly.)

Defined loosely as a push or a pull, a force is measured in pounds (lb, in the US customary system of units) or Newtons (N, in the Système International d'Unités [SI] system) (1 lb = 4.448 N). In general, force is a *vector* quantity, which means that its complete definition includes specifying both magnitude and direction. While the size (or *magnitude*) of a force may be expressed in units of lb or N, the magnitude alone is not a complete description of the force because, in general, it is also important to know the direction in which the force is acting. For example, a 10-lb force acting downward on a tooth or implant does not have the same effect as a 10-lb force acting sideways. (In contrast to a vector quantity, a *scalar* quantity—such as temperature, humidity, or density—is fully characterized by magnitude alone.)

There are various ways of denoting vectors in mechanics. For the purposes of illustrating forces in diagrams, a force vector is usually represented as an arrow, with the arrow's direction showing the direction in which the force acts. This direction is called the *line of action*. In dealing with forces and how they affect structures—in particular teeth, implants, and dentures—it is also important to specify the *point* at which the vector acts. Vectors are usually written in boldface (**F**) or with a line over them ($\bar{F}$). The magnitude of the vector is indicated in roman type (F).

Another important concept is the idea of *resolving a force vector into components* (Fig 6-2). As in the figure, let us assume that a force F arises because of point-contact between a small spherical particle of food and the surface of a crown during chewing. Furthermore, suppose that the crown is supported by a single underlying implant. Note in the diagram that the force does not act in a direction parallel to the axis of the implant; suppose the force acts at point B on the central axis of the implant. The question arises: What part of the applied force acts parallel to, and what part acts perpendicular to, the axis of the implant? (For instance, this question is relevant in the case where an implant or some part of it might fracture if the perpendicular component becomes too large.) A way to analyze this problem is to resolve the force vector into components along the directions of interest. To do this, a coordinate system is selected with x-, y-, and z-axes at right angles to one another (a so-called Cartesian coordinate system), with the z-axis parallel to the long axis of the implant, as shown in the diagram. Then, by considering

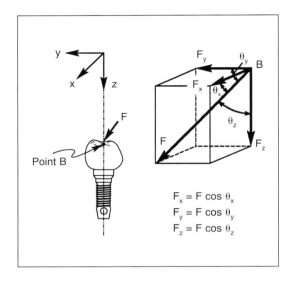

$$F_x = F \cos \theta_x$$
$$F_y = F \cos \theta_y$$
$$F_z = F \cos \theta_z$$

Fig 6-2 Force F acting at point B on the crown may be resolved into components directed along the x-, y-, and z-axes. (Reprinted from Naert et al[13] with permission.)

the angles that the force vector makes with the three coordinate axes, it is possible to resolve the force into its three components: F_z (acting along the z-axis) and lateral components F_x and F_y (acting along the x- and y-axes). The components of F are defined and computed by the following equations:

(1) $\qquad F_x = F \cos \theta_x$
(2) $\qquad F_y = F \cos \theta_y$
(3) $\qquad F_z = F \cos \theta_z$

In these equations, F is the scalar magnitude of the force. The angles θ_x, θ_y, and θ_z are the angles between the force vector and the x-, y-, and z-axes, respectively. For the sake of completeness, note that a useful relationship exists between the magnitude of the force (F) and the values of its three components:

(4) $\qquad F = \sqrt{F_x^2 + F_y^2 + F_z^2}$

Equation 4 follows from the definitions (equations 1, 2, and 3) and a known geo-

metric relationship among the three angles, namely:

(5) $\qquad \cos^2 \theta_x + \cos^2 \theta_y + \cos^2 \theta_z = 1$

As suggested here, the intuition that chewing forces always act parallel to the long axes of teeth and implants is an oversimplification. While it is ordinarily true that the largest component is the vertical force component, the vertical component is not necessarily the only component; it depends also on the facets and inclines on the surface of the crown or prosthesis.

Moments (torques)

Another essential concept from elementary mechanics is the idea of a *moment*, or *torque*. A moment or torque is a loading action that tends to rotate a body. Most commonly, moments on a body such as an implant or a tooth are produced by the actions of forces, which seems to beg the question of why there is a need for the concept of moments

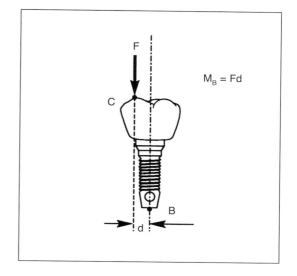

$$M_B = Fd$$

Fig 6-3 Example of a moment being produced on an implant as a result of so-called eccentric loading: The point at which the force is applied (C) is at a distance d from the center line of the implant, so the moment at a chosen point B is Fd, where d is the perpendicular distance from point B to the line of action of F. (Reprinted from Naert et al[13] with permission.)

in the first place. The explanation is that moments are inherent in the definition of equilibrium of a rigid body, ie, for static equilibrium of a rigid body, the sum of forces must be zero *along with the sum of the moments about any point.* So moments are inherent in defining equilibrium. (Another reason for introducing moments is that they are meaningful in analyses of stress and material failure, although this topic is beyond the scope of this chapter.) The dimensions of a moment are force multiplied by distance; hence, typical units are N m or N cm in the SI system and lb-ft or oz-in in the English system.

Examples of moments arise in many common situations. One example is the use of an ordinary screwdriver; here the hand supplies two things: *(1)* a pair of equal and opposite forces (called a *couple* or *couple-moment*) to the screwdriver handle, which tends to turn the screwdriver; and *(2)* a small axial "pushing" force, which is directed along the axis of the screwdriver. Strictly speaking, (1) and (2) together make up a resultant loading that is called a *wrench*—which supports the idea

that a screwdriver is actually a type of wrench. However, a focus on the torquing action on the screwdriver's handle—that couple, or couple-moment—provides a good example of a *moment,* or *torque,* about the axis of the screwdriver. A similar situation arises when one uses a torque wrench with a handle; here, the torque about the axis of the screw or nut that is being turned is created by a force on the handle multiplied by the perpendicular distance from the line of action of the force to the axis of the screw. As with the screwdriver, the resultant loading at the screw is made up of both a force and a moment. In a more clinically relevant example, consider one implant supporting a single crown that is loaded vertically, parallel to the long axis of the implant, but at a point C that is not on the center line of the implant (Fig 6-3). Here, by the rules of mechanics, at a point of interest such as the base of the implant near point B, the net (or resultant) loading at that point will consist of a moment equal to the magnitude of the force times the perpendicular distance between the line of action of the force and the implant's center line (eg, $M_B = Fd$), as well as the applied force F on the implant. For example, a moderate bite force of, say, 400 N, applied at a point on the crown that is 2 mm from the center line of the implant would produce (at point B, and also at any point along the center line of the implant) a resultant loading consisting of a force equal to 400 N and a moment equal to 400 N × 2 mm = 800 N mm = 80 N cm. To illustrate the significance of this magnitude of the moment, if one tried to use a traditional Brånemark System abutment (Nobel Biocare, Yorba Linda, CA) plus gold cylinder and gold screw to serve as a single-tooth prosthesis—which, of course, is not standard practice—then this level of moment (80 N cm) would be so large as to cause yielding of the screw joint.[14]

Although in formal mechanics a moment is a vector quantity, it serves our purposes here to simply speak of the moment about a point as being a scalar quantity equal to the force times the perpendicular distance between the point and the force's line of action. However, as with any vector, a moment can be resolved into three Cartesian components along the axes of a three-dimensional (3D) coordinate system. Referring back to an implant as a fixed support, Fig 6-1 illustrates that in the most general case, there can be three force components and three moment components—or a total of six loading components—acting on a fixed support. The goal of oral biomechanics is therefore twofold: *(1)* predict the typical values of these components when implants are subjected to typical use in vivo, and *(2)* evaluate whether these applied loading components are safe or dangerous.

Values of biting forces in vivo

Patients with no dental implants or dentures, and with healthy opposing natural teeth, can typically exert axial components of biting force in the range of 100 to 2,400 N, which is 27 to 550 lbs in English units (Table 6-1). However, exact bite force values depend on factors such as location in the mouth, nature of the food, chewing versus swallowing, degree of exertion by the patient, and presence or absence of parafunctional habits of the patient. In any case, the term *axial* refers to the force component acting parallel to the long axis of a natural tooth or implant, as discussed previously. (Sometimes the terms *vertical* or *occlusoapical* are used synonymously with *axial*.) Axial force components on natural teeth tend to be larger at more distal locations in the mouth. This is explained by an approximate model of the mandible as a class 3 lever, in which all forces—ie, those resulting from biting, joint reaction force at the temporomandibular joint (TMJ), and jaw muscle forces—are assumed to act in the sagittal plane (Fig 6-4). Moreover, assume that the lines of action of the forces resulting from the main muscles of mastication are distal to the point where the bite force typically occurs, and that the fulcrum of the lever is at the TMJ (point C in the diagram). This forms a class 3 lever with a mechanical advantage of less than one; the bite force will be larger if it acts nearer to the fulcrum, toward the TMJ.

Typical magnitudes of axial forces on natural teeth during mastication are available from many sources (see Table 6-1). These data should be regarded only as rough estimates for the typical magnitudes of axial forces on natural teeth in humans. The main limitation of these data is that the experimental techniques by which they

Table 6-1 Bite forces and related data

Description of data	Typical values
Vertical component of biting force in adults, averaged over several teeth[15]	200–2,440 N
Vertical component of biting force in adults, molar region[15]	390–880 N
Vertical component of biting force in adults, premolar region[15]	453 N
Vertical component of biting force in adults, incisor region[15]	222 N
Vertical component of biting force in adults wearing complete dentures[16–19]	77–196 N
Vertical component of biting force in adults with a maxillary denture opposed by natural teeth in mandible[16]	147–284 N
Vertical component of biting force in adults with dentures supported by implants (patients asked to exert maximum force)[20]	42–412 N (median 143 N)
Vertical component of biting force in adults with dentures supported by overdenture attachments[16]	337–342 N
Lateral components of bite forces in adults[21]	20 N (approx)
Frequency of chewing strokes[22]	60–80 strokes/min
Rate of chewing[21,23]	1–2 strokes/s
Duration of tooth contact in one chewing cycle[21]	0.23–0.3 s
Total time of tooth contact in a 24-hour period[21]	9–17.5 min
Maximum closure speed of jaws during chewing[22]	140 mm/s
Maximum contact stresses on teeth[24]	20 MPa

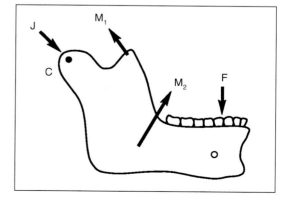

Fig 6-4 Simplified model of the jaw as a class 3 lever. The fulcrum is at the condyle (C), while the two major muscle forces (M_1 and M_2) act nearer to the fulcrum than the biting force F. J = joint reaction force. (Reprinted from Naert et al[13] with permission.)

were obtained involved the use of relatively large measuring devices, such as bite forks or bite wafers. Such devices sometimes interfere with and change the details of chewing so that the resulting data do not necessarily pertain to natural chewing events. Accordingly, data in Table 6-1 represent what might best be termed *closure forces*, ie, forces exerted on an object when the patient closes the teeth on the object. A closure force would tend to be axially directed, but its point of action and line of action can be uncertain in these types of experimental measurements. The uncertainty arises because the bite force transducer is sometimes so large that more than one tooth is involved in the biting event; consequently, there are a few points of contact (not just one) at which forces are acting. At a minimum, the data in Table 6-1 provide reasonable estimates of the magnitudes of expected biting forces in vivo.

Data on the lateral force components in the natural or restored human dentition are scarce (see Table 6-1). One study reported that typical lateral components were about 20 N, for the special case of a prosthesis in the first mandibular molar region. This magnitude appears small compared to typical axial force components in Table 6-1. In view of the earlier discussion on resolving forces into axial and lateral components and the influence of the curved surfaces of teeth, it is likely that the lateral components could exceed 20 N. For instance, a bite force of 200 N acting at 45 degrees to the long axis of an implant would have a purely lateral component equal to 141 N ($= 200$ N $\times$ cos 45°). So for design purposes with implants, for instance, it is prudent to consider whether the bending strength of an implant will be sufficient to withstand a lateral force of, say, 141 N.

Common personal experience shows that biting is a dynamic (time-varying) process rather than a static event. Table 6-1 shows that the maximum closure speed of the mandible relative to the maxilla is estimated at about 140 mm/s. While this seems like a moderately fast speed, nevertheless, a working assumption of most analyses is that dynamics and related inertial effects are not significant at such closing speeds and do not appreciably affect biting loads. This means that analyses based on statics alone appear to be sufficient for most purposes.

The net "chewing time per meal" has been found to be about 450 seconds. If the chewing frequency is about 1 Hz with a 0.3-second duration of tooth contact during each chewing stroke, there will be about 9 minutes per day during which chewing forces will act on teeth. If other activities such as swallowing are considered, the time might increase to about 17.5 minutes per day. Parafunctional habits such as bruxism could significantly increase this time. These estimates provide a useful indication of the minimum daily time per day that teeth (and perhaps implants) are load-bearing because of mastication and related events.

For the restored dentition (see Table 6-1), completely edentulous patients who have soft tissue–supported dentures in both arches tend to bite with about one-sixth less axial force than patients with natural teeth or a denture opposing natural teeth. While individuals wearing complete maxillary and/or mandibular dentures have often shown an impaired ability to bite on solid objects, it can be possible for them to exert higher local loading levels than dentate patients if there is a balanced support of the denture.

For edentulous patients restored with full-arch prostheses supported by dental implants, axial closure forces have been shown to be approximately equal to the forces in the normal dentate patient (see Table 6-1).

Values of moments in vivo

Moments develop on implants largely from the action of forces, as noted earlier. As with forces, it is important to distinguish among different possible components of a moment, for instance, moment components about the x-, y-, and z-axes of the fixed support idealization (see Fig 6-1). Unfortunately, there have been few studies to determine typical values of moments applied to implants in vivo in various sorts of clinical situations. From direct measurements by several groups working with human subjects who had implants[25–29] and from simulations with finite element models,[30,31] it is known that typical values of the buccolingual and mesiodistal bending moments can be in the range of 0 to 40 N cm, with maximal values estimated in computer models as large as 70 N cm. Values for the moment component about the long axis of an implant are on the order of 10 N cm. Pending more extensive data and better estimates for how values depend upon prosthesis design and other factors, these data at least serve as a guide to expected moments.

Prediction of Forces and Moments on Dental Implants

The problem and an introductory solution

Assuming that the biting forces on a prosthesis are known, the problem is how to compute the loadings on multiple supporting abutments (natural teeth or implants). In general, for a multi-abutment case, the force on an abutment will not be the same as the bite force exerted on the prosthesis. A simple first example makes this clear. Suppose a downward force P acts at the end of an implant prosthesis with a cantilever section (Fig 6-5). The distance between the line of action of P and the nearest implant (#2 in Fig 6-5) is a, the length of the cantilever portion of the prosthesis. The prosthesis is assumed to be a rigid (undeformable) body supported by two implants (#1 and #2) that are spaced b apart. The problem is to predict the forces on implants #1 and #2.

In the simplest analysis, we employ a model involving rigid-body static equilibrium in two dimensions (2D). The analysis begins with a so-called *free-body diagram* of the prosthesis, which is drawn as a simple beam in Fig 6-5. The beam is isolated (removed from the implants), and all forces acting on the beam are shown. (The beam is assumed to have no appreciable weight.) Forces F_1 and F_2 represent the forces that the implants exert on the beam. The true directions of the forces do not have to be known at this stage of the analysis; the correct directions will emerge from the solution. (However, in this example the forces act in the correct directions.) The assumption that only forces—and no moments—exist at the prosthesis-implant connection(s) comes from the idealization that the implants are connected to the prosthesis by pin joints in this 2D model; pin joints transmit only force components and not moments. (In the 3D analog of this example, a ball-and-socket joint would be the comparable connection.) Force P is the biting force. The next step is to recognize that the beam is in static equilibrium, which means, according to Newton's laws, that

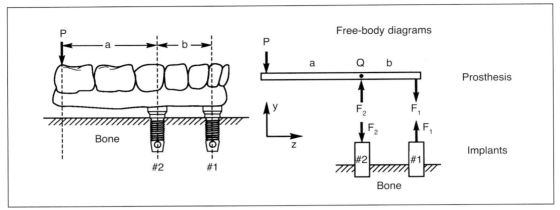

Fig 6-5 A method for predicting the forces on two implants supporting a cantilever portion of a prosthesis. *(left)* A diagrammatic view of the situation in 2D. *(right)* Free-body diagrams of the prosthesis *(top)* and the implants *(bottom)*. P = biting force; Q = point at which summation of moments is being found. (Reprinted from Naert et al[13] with permission.)

the sum of the forces and the sum of the moments on the beam must equal zero. The application of equilibrium allows us to solve for the two unknown forces F_1 and F_2; this is done by solving the two equations of static equilibrium (note sign conventions according to the coordinate system in Fig 6-5):

$$(6) \qquad \Sigma F_y = 0: -F_1 + F_2 - P = 0$$
$$\Sigma M_Q = 0: -F_1 b + aP = 0$$

The notation ΣF_y means summation of forces in the y-direction, while ΣM_Q means summation of moments about point Q. (Q is not unique; any point could have been chosen with the same final result.) The solution of these two equations in two unknowns is

$$(7) \qquad F_2 = (1+a/b)P \text{ and } F_1 = (a/b)P$$

The above analysis has important ramifications. First, it shows that although the prosthesis is loaded by a biting force P, the implants are loaded by forces whose magnitudes can be larger than P, depending on the ratio a/b. That is, for a/b = 2, which is not an uncommon value in clinical practice, the forces on the implants will be 3P and 2P. In understanding the directions in which these forces act, note that the forces on the prosthesis from the implants are equal but opposite to the forces on the implants from the prosthesis; this arises from Newton's third law, ie, for every action there is an equal and opposite reaction. Also note that forces F_1 and F_2 do not act in the same direction; implant #2, nearest to the point at which P acts, experiences a compressive load, tending to push it into the bone, while implant #1 experiences a tensile load, tending to pull it out of the bone. So the key result from this introductory analysis is that the loading on the implant(s) can exceed the loading on the prosthesis.

A numeric example based on the above helps drive home the point. Consider a moderately low level of typical biting force

P, eg, 250 N, and select a reasonable a/b ratio of 2; then the tensile force on implant #1 will be 2P = 2 × 250 N = 500 N, while the compressive force on implant #2 is 3P = 3 × 250 N = 750 N. As a quick indication of the possible clinical significance of such force levels on dental implants, it is known that implant loadings of 250 to 500 N can exceed the failure strength of many implants that have been tested in various animal models. For example, to cite just two examples of data, Block and Kent[32] measured maximal pullout strengths of about 150 N for hydroxyapatite (HA)-coated cylindrical implants that had healed in dog mandibles for 32 weeks, while Burgess et al[33] measured mean pullout forces of about 200 to 350 N at 3 weeks and 15 weeks, respectively, after placing cylindrical HA-coated implants in dog bone. Of course, many factors influence the strength of the bone-implant interface, including healing time, cancellous versus cortical bone site, and size and shape of the implant.[1] Unfortunately, for human cases, the field does not yet have an extensive database of strengths of bone-implant interfaces for various implants in different types of bone quality and quantity, even though this database is part of what is needed to establish safe versus dangerous applied force levels on implants.

More complicated prosthetic situations and biomechanical models

As noted in the previous section, the two-implant case is not the general case of implant use, nor is it necessarily true that implants are connected to a perfectly rigid prosthesis with pin or ball-and-socket joints. In general, there is a need to be able to compute the expected forces and moments on more than two implant abutments supporting a loaded prosthesis of arbitrary shape, size, and material that is screwed, cemented, or otherwise attached to the implant abutments. A number of complicating factors can arise in trying to solve this more general case, including:

- Full or partial prosthesis
- Number and location of implant (and/or natural tooth) abutments
- Angulations of the implants
- Nature of the prosthesis-abutment connection
- Use of overdentures supported by a mixture of soft tissue and implants
- Mechanical properties of the material(s) and structure of the prosthesis, implants, and bone (eg, elastic moduli, structural stiffnesses)
- Deformability of the mandible or maxilla
- Misfit of the prosthesis relative to the supporting implants

Biomechanical models that account for some of these factors are discussed here, with examples to illustrate how the models work. Generally, these models fall into two broad categories. One category consists of analytic models, eg, models that provide closed-form (explicit) equations allowing calculation of the forces and moments on the implants; these analytic models can typically be solved with pencil and paper, pocket calculator, or personal computer. A good example is the Skalak model from the early 1980s.[34] A second category of model consists of more complicated computer models, eg, finite element (FE) models. Although some FE models can run on ordinary personal computers, the more involved FE models require the use of sophisticated, proprietary, high-end software running on workstations. Ideally, such FE models should only be used by operators with a reasonably advanced understanding of solid mechanics and stress analysis.

Whatever the model, the most important point is that both analytic and computer models are indeed models, or idealizations, of reality. As such, some models may come closer to reality than others. Whether one analytic method is "better" than another does not depend on the inherent complexity of the model as much as it depends on the goals of the analysis and the assumptions that go into the model; a simple model used properly is superior to a complex model used without an understanding of its limitations. In general, the best advice is that a clinician must understand the underlying assumptions and methods of a particular model in relation to reality. Also, to gain confidence in a model, at some point it is essential to check how the model's predictions stack up against reality.

Approximate model for fully edentulous cases

For a fully edentulous case involving, for example, four maxillary implants supporting a maxillary prosthesis (Fig 6-6), a highly simplified model proposed by Rangert et al[14] can be used as a quick estimate of implant loading. This model considers only the pair of implants closest to the applied bite force as the "active" (loaded) pair of implants. The distances a and b in Fig 6-6 could be measured, along with an estimate of the biting force at a location of interest, eg, at the end of the cantilever. The forces on the two implants nearest to the bite force could be obtained by the same 2D methods outlined previously, where the forces on the two implants depend on the bite force P and the ratio a/b. In a sense, the simple approach of

Rangert et al[14] converts a 3D problem into a easily solvable 2D model. However, the obvious limitation of this approach is that it does not account for loading of all four implants in the sketch; the model assumes that only the two implants nearest the applied bite force are "doing all the work." In reality, this is incorrect and cannot be expected to give an accurate estimate of implant loading in all multi-implant cases. However, this approach does provide a quick, first-order estimate of the loading of the two implants nearest to an end-loaded cantilever of a prosthesis.

Skalak model for cases involving three or more implants

In the language of mechanics, the problem of predicting loads on all implant abutments in a multi-implant distribution is a statically indeterminate problem. This means that the abutment loadings cannot be obtained using only the theory of rigid-body statics (ie, the underlying theory of the previous examples in this chapter). However, it is possible to solve a statically indeterminate problem if additional information is available, such as in the model presented by Skalak in the early 1980s.[34]

Skalak's model was based on an established method in mechanical engineering for predicting the load distribution among bolts or rivets joining rigid plates. When applied to the oral implant situation, this approach idealizes the prosthesis and the jaw as two rigid "plates" joined by spring-like bolts; the model predicts the vertical and horizontal force components on spring-like implants supporting a prosthesis (plate) subjected to vertical and horizontal loadings (Fig 6-7). Essentially, the model assumes that the implants are elastic springs with known spring constants. The detailed equa-

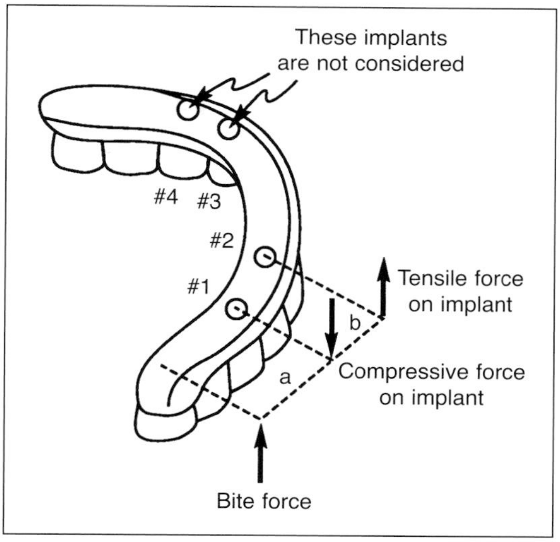

These implants
are not considered

#4 #3

#2

#1

Tensile force
on implant

b

a

Compressive force
on implant

Bite force

Fig 6-6 Diagrammatic view of a maxillary prosthesis loaded by a bite force. Forces at implant locations #1 and #2 can be predicted approximately by the same method used in Fig 6-5, provided that implants at locations #3 and #4 are assumed not to participate. (Reprinted from Naert et al[13] with permission.)

tions for the model are given in the figure; the main finding is that a purely vertical force on the prosthesis (ie, acting perpendicular to the plane of the prosthesis) is counterbalanced by a distribution of purely vertical forces among the number of (N) supporting abutments. Similarly, for a horizontal load on the prosthesis (ie, acting in the plane of the prosthesis), the model predicts that there will be a counterbalancing distribution of horizontal forces among the N abutments. (The model breaks down for fewer than three implants because ball-and-socket connections are assumed where the springs meet the prosthesis.) In the general case of an arbitrary force vector on the prosthesis, with both vertical and horizontal components, the resultant loading on each implant is the combined result of the vertical and horizontal load components, which can be computed independent of one another. Likewise, if there are several points at

which forces are applied to the prosthesis, the model can be run for each of these situations independently, with the final loading on any one implant found by superposition of results from the various loading calculations. Shown next are some example results computed with the Skalak model; they illustrate its usefulness as well as the key fact that implant loading can vary as a function of various factors, eg, number of implants, their locations, and their arrangement relative to one another.

Example 1: Four versus six implants

Consider two cases first: four or six implants symmetrically distributed about the midline of a mandible over the same arc of 112.5 degrees, with the radius of the mandible equal to 22.5 mm (Fig 6-8). The arc of 112.5 degrees represents a distance roughly equal to that between the mental foramina in the human mandible. The Skalak model is used

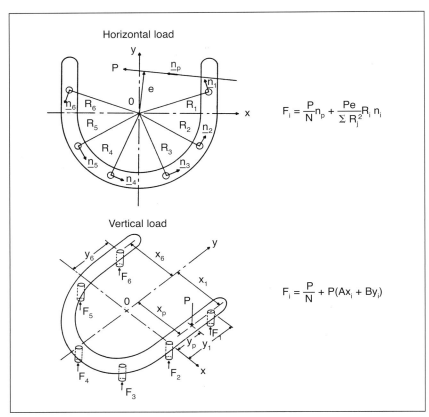

Horizontal load

$$F_i = \frac{P}{N}n_p + \frac{Pe}{\Sigma R_j^2}R_i\, n_i$$

Vertical load

$$F_i = \frac{P}{N} + P(Ax_i + By_i)$$

Fig 6-7 The Skalak (1983) model.[34] Given the number, N, and arrangement of the implants, the horizontal and vertical forces on each implant can be computed using the equations shown under either horizontal or vertical loading by force P. For further explanation of terms in the equations, see Brunski[35] and Brunski and Skalak.[36] (Reprinted from Naert et al[13] with permission.)

to predict the vertical forces on each implant when a single vertical force of magnitude 30 N acts at a position defined by $\theta =$ 10 degrees. Note first that for a six-implant case with a vertical load of 30 N at $\theta = 10$ degrees (a case of cantilever loading), the most distal implants nearest the load (#1 and #2) experience compressive forces (negative values) as does implant #6, on the other side of the prosthesis. Meanwhile, the three anterior implants (#3, #4, and #5) experience tensile forces (positive values). This result can be understood by recognizing that the implants are exerting forces on the prosthesis to keep it from tipping distally and to the side under the action of the applied cantilever loading. Note also that for the applied vertical load magnitude of 30 N, the loads on the implants are less than 30 N except for the load on implant #1 nearest the loading point, which is about −40 N (the negative sign indicates compression).

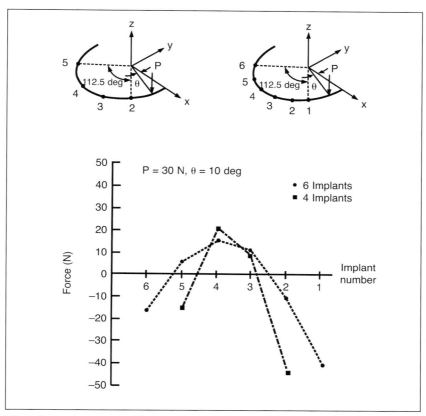

Fig 6-8 Results from the Skalak model for a four- versus a six-implant case when the implants span the same arc (112.5 degrees). The four-implant case has a larger interimplant spacing than the six-implant case. The graph shows that the implant force levels are not dramatically different in the six-implant versus the four-implant case. (Reprinted from Naert et al[13] with permission.)

Now, to compare the case above with a four-implant case, consider the results *when four implants are spaced out over the same arc as the six-implant case above (112.5 degrees)*, per Fig 6-8. What happens is that the magnitudes of the forces on the most distal implants are similar in both the four- and six-implant cases. In other words, there is only a slight difference between using four implants and using six implants to support a prosthesis, at least for this case, when the

four implants are spaced out over the same arc as the six implants. The explanation for this resides largely in the fact that the interimplant spacing in the four-implant case is larger than that in the six-implant case; this compensates for fewer implants, which would otherwise tend to increase the loading per implant (as seen in the following paragraph). Generally consistent with this analysis, 10-year clinical studies with the Brånemark System in full-arch cases indi-

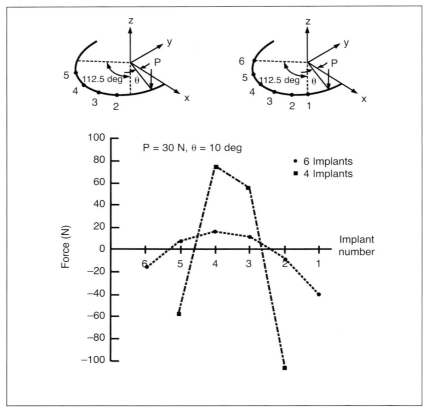

Fig 6-9 Results from the Skalak model for a four- versus six-implant case in which the four implants do not span the same arc as the six implants (112.5 degrees). The graph shows that the forces on the implants are much larger in the four-implant case. (Reprinted from Naert et al[13] with permission.)

cated that prostheses supported by four implants did just as well as those supported by six implants.[37]

In contrast, consider now a new arrangement of four implants created by removing the two most distal implants (#1 and #6) from the six-implant case analyzed above, but this time keeping the interimplant spacing the same as it was in the six-implant case. Now the forces on the four remaining implants become markedly larger than in the original six-implant case (Fig 6-9). Taking this a step farther, an even worse situation would consist of four implants positioned in a straight-line arrangement (rather than in a curved arc) across the anterior of the mandible; this results in even larger forces per implant when the prosthesis is loaded by a vertical force in the distal cantilever region.

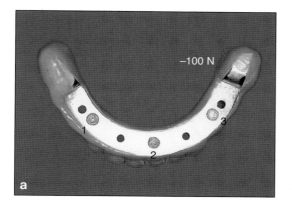

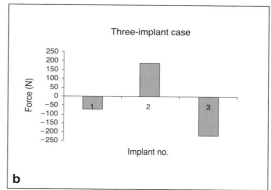

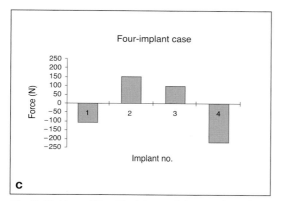

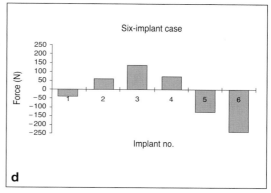

Fig 6-10 Use of the Skalak model to explore the loading per implant when three, four, or six implants are spread out along the same arc as used in the new Brånemark Novum System. *(a)* A downward bite force of −100 N is applied at the same cantilever region in each case. (Reprinted from Vasconcelos and Franischone[40] with permission.) *(b–d)* Predicted axial forces on the implants. While the implant forces are a bit greater in the three-implant case, the differences among the three situations are not dramatic.

Example 2: The new three-implant Novum System

An interesting case arises with the newly developed Brånemark Novum System (Nobel Biocare) for immediate loading,[38,39] which uses only three implants in the anterior mandible for immediate support of a specially designed prosthesis attached on the same day as the implant placement surgery. The three implants in this system resemble the typical pure titanium, 3.75-mm-diameter screws of the conventional Brånemark System but have a larger diameter of 5 mm. Part of the biomechanical rationale behind the performance of this system can be understood by applying the 1983 Skalak model,[34] as illustrated in Fig 6-10. Here, three cases are compared in which there are three, four, or six implants spaced out along the same arc length in the anterior of the mandible.

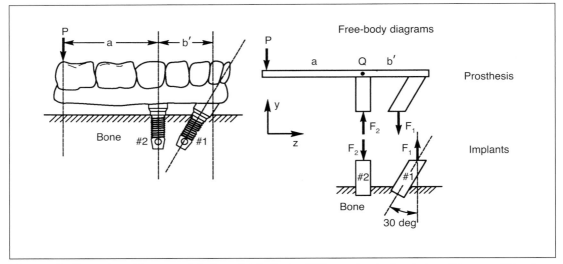

Fig 6-11 An illustration of the potentially beneficial effects of tilting an implant; note how this case differs from that in Fig 6-5; b′ > b, which affects the force levels on implants #1 and #2 relative to the results from Fig 6-5. (Reprinted from Naert et al[13] with permission.)

For comparison purposes, only one loading condition of the prosthesis is examined, namely, that of a vertical force of –100 N applied at the distal cantilever region. A comparison of the results from the three cases illustrates that although there are some differences in the cases, these differences are relatively minor in terms of the overall magnitude of loading per implant. For example, while the maximum tensile load on any implant is indeed larger in the three- and four-implant cases than in the six-implant case, the maximal values are within only a few percent of one another. In addition, even though the tensile force is a bit larger in the three-implant case, the 5-mm implant diameter of the Novum implant would tend to decrease bone stresses as a result of the increased implant area, which may offset the somewhat larger tensile force in the three-implant Novum case. Detailed analysis of this system has not yet been pro-

vided, but nevertheless the Skalak model analysis already allows one to grasp the essential design rationale of the Novum System, which is that three larger-diameter implants can, in principle, serve the purpose of four or six implants, especially if the three implants are spaced out along the same arc length that would have been occupied by four or six implants.

Another issue that arises in immediate loading is the stiffness of the implants in the bone: Is the stiffness of the implant in bone the same at each location at the time of implant placement? This can be a factor in the load distribution, as discussed in the next section of this chapter. Another factor is the rigidity of the prosthesis, which is also discussed later on.

Example 3: Use of angulated implants
Another new clinical development that can be understood on the basis of analysis with

Fig 6-12 Illustration of numeric changes in the forces on three implants when the distal implant is tilted by a few millimeters toward the distal and the prosthesis is loaded at the end of a cantilever. *(a)* The numbers in the parentheses are x,y coordinates of the implants and applied force, in image units. These data are used in the Skalak model along with the bite force. *(b)* Case A: Implant #1 is upright. *(c)* Case B: Implant #1 is tilted. The Skalak model predicts a decrease in maximal force levels by at least 50% relative to case A.

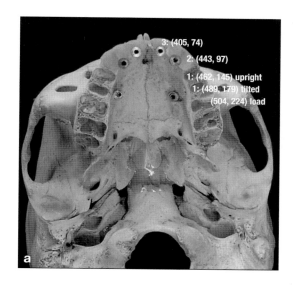

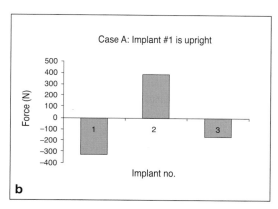

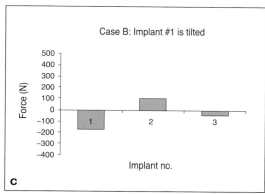

the Skalak model is the use of angulated implants. It has been proposed that angled implants can help support prostheses in partially edentulous cases, eg, as in the studies of Krekmanov et al.[41] Starting with the simplest case, consider a partially edentulous case having a slight cantilever in the bridge and resembling the earlier example in Fig 6-5, except that here implant #1 is inclined to the vertical by 30 degrees (Fig 6-11). The solution to the force distribution problem (see equation 7) now has one difference in

this case: at the points of contact with the prosthesis, the interimplant spacing increases from b to b' as a result of the tilting. So now for the same applied load (P) and cantilever distance (a), it follows from equation 7 and b' > b that the forces on implants #1 and #2 will decrease relative to what they were when implant #1 was upright.

We can explore numeric changes in the forces by using the Skalak model applied to a case with dimensions taken from an actual skull (Fig 6-12). We compute the load distribution among three implants supporting a partial prosthesis in the maxilla. In case A, all three implants are upright and perpendicular to the plane of the prosthesis, with implant #1 located back toward the distal end of a cantilever that is end-loaded by a force of –100 N, which is directed upward (toward the cranium). Alternatively, case B has implant #1 slightly tilted to the distal, so that it connects to the prosthesis at a point located a few millimeters more distal than in case A. Analysis of these two cases with the Skalak model reveals that the forces on implants #1, #2, and #3 in case B are appreciably decreased relative to case A because of the tilting of implant #1.

Now, one might object that this analysis does not consider the stress-strain patterns in the bone in case A versus case B and that these stress patterns might be more severe around the tilted versus the upright implant even if the force on the tilted implant has decreased relative to when it was straight. Indeed, it is expected that for the same force on an upright versus an inclined implant (with all else being equal), there would tend to be higher stresses and strains in bone around the tilted implant.[42] However, the advantages of the tilting are that (1) it decreases the forces on all of the implants by redistributing the loading, and (2) a lower force on the tilted implant could offset an increase in stresses and strains in bone (and implant parts) that would otherwise tend to occur because of the tilting. This subject is still under clinical study, but, again, this analysis with the original Skalak model[34] can provide some insight into the basic biomechanical principles that are involved.

Additional Factors in the Prediction of Implant Loading

Implant stiffness

The stiffness of an implant (or a natural tooth, for that matter) is related to the clinical term *mobility*. Here, the word *mobility* does not mean orthodontically induced movement resulting from biologic activities around a tooth or implant. Instead it means relatively small (eg, tenths to thousandths of a millimeter) and reversible displacements of teeth or implants caused by temporarily applied forces. At the clinical level, mobility describes tooth or implant movement in axial or lateral directions with respect to a fixed reference, eg, fixed bone in the rest of the jaw. When testing tooth mobility, a dentist typically applies a lateral force to a tooth with a dental instrument (say a mirror handle) and then estimates the lateral movement of the tooth with the naked eye. While movements greater than, eg, 1 mm are easily detected and would suggest an advanced degree of breakdown in periodontal support, movements of, eg, 0.020 mm (20 μm) would be imperceptible to the naked eye. However, such small movement can be mechanically important nonetheless, especially when it comes to predicting how implants (and teeth) behave when splinted together in supporting a prosthesis.

For example, in the case of a prosthesis supported by both teeth and implants, complications arise in predicting the load sharing among the abutments. The complications arise because natural teeth and implants do not have the same mobility characteristics, which is known from direct measurements (Table 6-2). Moreover, some

Table 6-2 Data on intrusive stiffness of dental implants and teeth

Implant or tooth	Stiffness (N/μm)
IMZ implant (Interpore International, Irvine, CA) with intramobile element (IME), transmucosal implant extension (TIE), and gold screw[43]	2.57
Flexiroot implant (Facial Alveodental Implant Rehabilitation, Bala Cynwyd, PA) with polymer insert and attachment (per A. Haris)[43]	4.11
Brånemark implant (7 mm) plus abutment screw, abutment, and gold cylinder[43]	4.55
Driskell implant (Stryker, Kalamazoo, MI), with abutment (precursor to Bicon implant [Bicon, Boston, MA])[43]	5.50
Brånemark implant (7 mm) in trabecular bone (bovine tibial metaphysis)[43]	2.50
Brånemark implant in polycarbonate plastic[43]	3.66
Titanium blade-vent implant in fibrous tissue, retrieved sample from dog mandible[44]	0.22–0.88
Bioglass cylindrical implants in fibrous tissue, retrieved dog mandible[45]	1.9
Bioglass cylindrical implants with a direct bone-implant interface, retrieved dog mandible[45]	8.5
Tübingen Al_2O_3 implant in human mandible (in vivo)[46]	10*
Human molar (in vivo)[47]	0.1–1.0*
Human incisor (in vivo)[48]	0.1–3.0*
Human maxillary left first premolar (in vivo)[46]	0.1–1.0*

*Data estimated from slopes of graphs in publication.

researchers[49,50] suggest that the combination of implants with natural teeth seems to carry a greater rate of complications. Such studies point to differing mobility of teeth and implants as a causative factor in predisposing these cases to complications. However, so far in this chapter, none of the simple models for predicting abutment loading explicitly account for differing mobility among abutments. Fortunately, there is a modification to the Skalak model[51] that does consider differing abutment mobility, as discussed shortly. First, however, we must discuss some facts about tooth and implant mobility to help establish a definition of stiffness.

It is known that teeth and implants can displace intrusively, extrusively, buccolingually, and mesiodistally and that tooth displacements can occur in more than one direction even when the applied force only acts in one direction. (The last detail is a secondary complication that is ignored for our purposes herein.) Second, when a constant force is applied to a tooth or implant, the displacement of the tooth or implant may increase slowly with time; this phenomenon is called *creep*. With implants, creep is probably not significant unless there is fibrous tissue around the implant (see the references to Brunski and Schock[44] and Weinstein et al[45] in Table 6-2). Third, intrusive tooth displacement is not always linear with intrusive force; data for maxillary incisors show an approximately bilinear relationship between intrusive displacement and intrusive force on a tooth, with the tooth displacing less per unit load when loaded beyond about 49 N.

In defining stiffness, it is also necessary to more fully define tooth or implant *displacement*. Displacement is a vector quantity, having both magnitude and direction. For example, if one pushes laterally with a 1-N force on the tip of a tooth, the tip of the tooth might move (displace) 0.2 mm in a direction parallel to the applied force. Alternatively, a 1-N force in a different direction— say, downward, parallel to the tooth's long axis, ie, an intrusive force—might cause an intrusive displacement of 0.1 mm. In either case, a coordinate system is needed to describe both the force and displacement. Typically one picks an x-y-z coordinate system that is fixed with respect to some reference point, such as nearby jawbone. Now, although the literature data cited above on tooth and implant mobility show that they do not behave exactly like simple, linear springs, for present purposes this idealization (or model) is sufficient as an approximation. So here we can assume that when a force F is applied to a tooth or implant, the displacement from its equilibrium position, Δx, is related to the force by the following simple equation for a spring:

(8) $$F = k\Delta x$$

Here k is a spring constant, or *stiffness*, having the units of force/displacement (for example, N/mm or N/µm). The stiffness k de-

pends on the material and structural properties of the tooth or implant as well as the mechanical properties of the tissues supporting the tooth or implant. Assuming that the tooth or implant stiffness is one spring (with spring constant k_{tooth} or $k_{implant}$) attached in a series, with a second spring representing the tissue interface (with spring constant $k_{interface}$), then these two springs in series have the net spring constant, k_{net}, given by:

(9) $$1/k_{net} = 1/k_{implant} + 1/k_{interface}$$

Based on this idealization, Table 6-2 shows typical stiffness data for teeth and implants as estimated from test data reported in a variety of sources. Values of about 3 to 5 N/µm have been determined for the net spring stiffness of the older-style IMZ (pressfit) implant system (non-threaded and titanium-plasma-sprayed, or HA-coated), which involved a titanium implant with a deformable inner element called an intramobile element (IME) made of a polymer. Table 6-2 shows that most implants in bone are characterized by a net stiffness that is larger than that for natural teeth; in Table 6-2 the largest stiffness value of 10 N/µm is for an alumina implant in bone. However, if there is a soft tissue interface (fibrous nonosseointegrated interface) around an implant, then the stiffness values are lower than those of implants with an osseointegrated interface, with the former resembling the stiffness values of periodontally compromised natural teeth.

Based on this concept of stiffness, the problem of predicting the distribution of forces and moments among natural teeth and implants supporting a prosthesis can now be revisited. Experimentally, it has been observed (Figs 6-13a and 6-13b) that im-

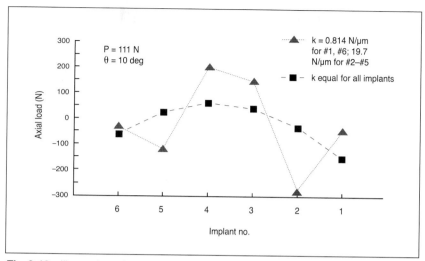

Fig 6-13a Illustration of changes in the forces among abutments when implants #1 and #6 have about a 10× lower stiffness (ie, are more compliant) than implants #2, #3, #4, and #5. The results are generated with the Skalak et al[51] model, which can account for differering stiffness among abutments. The effect of lower stiffness at #1 and #6 is an increase in the forces on implants #2, #3, #4 and #5, which in a sense converts a six-implant case into a four-implant case. (Reprinted from Brunski[52] with permission from Elsevier.)

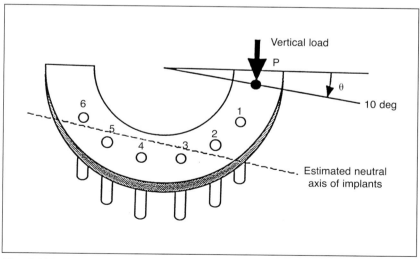

Fig 6-13b Perspective view of the loading situation analyzed in Fig 6-13a. (Reprinted from Brunski[52] with permission from Elsevier.)

plant stiffness is indeed important, eg, if low-stiffness abutments are located bilaterally at the two most distal locations in a six-implant distribution, then they support much less force—while the other four higher-stiffness implants support much larger forces—than in the case of a equal-stiffness implants in a six-implant case. In effect, when the two most distal implants are less stiff than the other four implants, a six-implant distribution is converted into a four-implant distribution. To incorporate stiffness into a Skalak-type model, one assumes or measures the axial and lateral stiffness of each implant and then uses that data in a modified version of the original Skalak model, ie, the 1993 Skalak et al model.[51] Results from this model show good agreement with data from laboratory testing (see Figs 6-13a and 6-13b). (This 1993 model was modified further by Brunski and Hurley[53] to incorporate work by Morgan and James,[54] which allowed for the support of a moment by the abutment-prosthesis joints.)

Deformability of the prosthesis

Analyses of forces and moments on implants supporting prostheses have also been accomplished by the FE modeling method. FE models allow the investigation of factors that cannot yet be easily addressed with analytic models, such as the mechanical properties of the prostheses, implants, and bone. Of course, as previously mentioned, these FE models can only be as good as the input data used to formulate them. While it is usually simple enough to obtain data about prostheses and implants, the problem is to obtain good data on exact properties for bone as it exists at interfaces of real implants and elsewhere in the jaw. As a rule, the output of most FE models has to

be viewed with awareness of the inherent limitations of the model—just as when any model is considered. Nevertheless, the FE models have been helpful in showing certain trends regarding the influence of the prosthesis.

For example, an FE model by Elias and Brunski[55]—together with laboratory testing and analytic modeling—leads to the conclusion that the structural rigidity of the prosthesis can affect the way that loading is shared among the abutments. For example, the load distribution among six implants did not exactly follow the predictions of the 1983 Skalak model[34] when the prosthesis was made out of either 100% acrylic or 100% casting alloy (Fig 6-14). With both the acrylic and the alloy, FE models and direct measurements of laboratory models showed that forces were more concentrated on those implants nearest to the loading point; for example, in Fig 6-14 note that implants #3, #4, #5, and #6 took hardly any load in the experiments and in the FE models; this differs from the predictions of the Skalak model. Evidently, neither the all-acrylic nor the metal frameworks were infinitely rigid, although the infinite-rigidity assumption is the inherent assumption of the 1983 Skalak model. The FE model more accurately reflects reality than does the Skalak model because the FE model accounts for the actual dimensions and material properties of the prosthesis. Other FE models of actual prostheses show the same trend as discussed above.[30,31,56] However, these FE studies did not give enough information to permit a one-to-one comparison of their results with predictions from the Skalak model.

In general, studies such as those cited above are needed to assess the role of the rigidity of actual prostheses as used by clinicians. Along these lines, direct testing of ex-

Fig 6-14 *(a)* A finite element (FE) model (Elias and Brunski[55]) used to predict forces on six implants supporting a full-arch prosthesis. The model is loaded with 35 N in the distal cantilever region. *(b and c)* Plots show axial forces on the implants when the prosthesis is metal *(b)* versus acrylic *(c)*. One line shows the predictions of an FE model (FEM), a second shows results measured directly using transducers in laboratory tests (experimental), and a third shows predictions of the Skalak model[33] (Skalak theory). Note that FE results match reality more closely than do those of the Skalak model, which assumes that the prosthesis is infinitely rigid. This work indicates that prosthesis rigidity does influence load sharing among abutments. (Reprinted from Naert et al[13] with permission.)

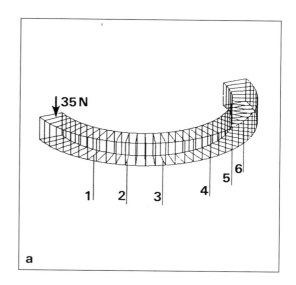

a

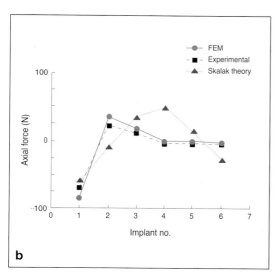

b

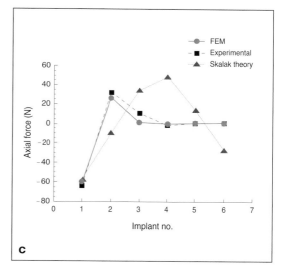

c

amples of clinical prostheses was conducted in the author's laboratory using three-point bending tests. The results showed that acrylic-veneered cast metal framework prostheses were slightly stiffer than all-acrylic prostheses in terms of the engineering property known as bending rigidity, which is the product of Young's elastic modulus (E) and the moment of inertia (I) of the prosthesis' cross section, *EI*. Results showed EI values for two clinically used, acrylic-veneered, cast metal framework prostheses of 0.91 ± 0.53 N m^2 and 0.57 ± 0.2 N m^2, while values for two similar-

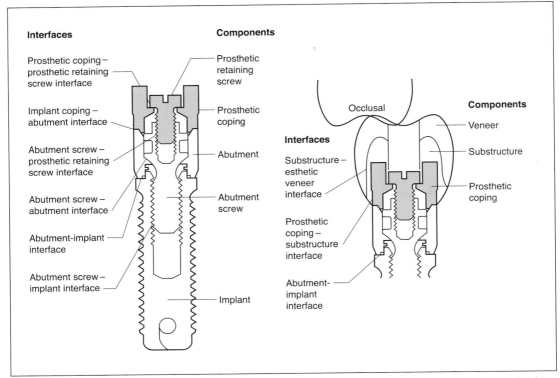

Fig 6-15 Diagrammatic cutaway view of the internal structure of the screw joints in the conventional Bråne-mark implant system.

sized, all-acrylic prostheses were 0.74 ± 0.47 N m² and 0.39 ± 0.06 N m². Interestingly, while there is perhaps a trend toward a larger *EI* with acrylic-veneered metal frame-work prostheses (as expected, because of the larger Young's modulus of cast metal versus acrylic), the EI values for the two types of frameworks were not markedly different. This point, taken together with the previous discussion of FE models and laboratory testing of load distributions among abutments supporting all-acrylic versus cast metal frameworks, supports the idea that neither all-acrylic nor all-metal frameworks are infinitely rigid in the sense assumed in the Skalak theory.

Frameworks, screw joints, and misfit

Another factor that can influence how implants are loaded is the quality of fit between the prosthesis and the implant abutments. In common implant systems, a metal framework of a full-arch or partial prosthesis is held onto the abutments by screw joints. For example, in the original Brånemark System, two screw joints exist. One screw joint's function is to clamp the gold cylinder (which is cast into the framework) to the abutment cylinder (Fig 6-15). But another joint exists where the abutment screw threads into the implant body to clamp the abutment cylinder to the implant. The biomechanics of both screw joints are important in determining the loading of the component parts of the implant system, which in turn influence the likelihood of problems and failure. Also, the screw joints play a role in misfit and in the implant loading that can occur as a result. This is explained after the following brief introduction to screw joint mechanics.

Screw joint mechanics

Basic principles of screw joints can be illustrated using the original Brånemark System. In this system, when the gold screw (also called the "prosthetic retaining screw" in Fig 6-15) is torqued into the abutment screw at the prescribed torque, that torque, T (which is nominally 10 N cm), induces a tensile force in the gold screw and a compressive clamping force at the interface of the gold cylinder (or "prosthetic coping" in Fig 6-15) and the abutment. The tensile force and the compressive force are equal and opposite and hold the screw joint closed. According to theory, the relationship between the torque T applied to the gold screw and the tensile force F that develops in the screw is given by the equation

(10) $$T = kDF$$

Here k is a dimensionless constant whose value depends on factors including screw thread geometry and friction at interfaces, and D is the screw diameter. Under ideal conditions in the original Brånemark System, an applied torque of 10 N cm on the gold screw produces a tensile force of about 300 N in the shaft of the flat-headed gold screw (and in the titanium abutment screw to which it is attached), and it induces an equal but opposite compressive force at the

interface of the gold cylinder and titanium abutment. The joint-clamping force, along with the tensile force in the gold screw, is often called the *preload* because it is the force set up within the joint before the abutment system is loaded by any external loading in the mouth. It is important to understand that the preload is an internal loading within the metallic pieces of the implant system; it causes no appreciable loading at the bone-implant interface.

The preload is quite significant, because a screw joint will start to open if the externally applied tensile force on the gold cylinder (eg, as applied by a loaded prosthesis that is attached to the gold cylinder) starts to exceed the force level of the preload in the screw joint system. (For a more exact discussion of the internal mechanics of screw joints, see the excellent discussion in Patterson and Johns[57]). Another important point about preload is that the 300-N preload claimed for the standard Brånemark System pertains only to ideal conditions in the Brånemark gold screw joint. Nonideal conditions in that joint can change the preload value appreciably. Examples of nonideal conditions in the gold screw joint (which apply also to the abutment screw joint) include uneven, pitted, or damaged mating surfaces between the gold screw and gold cylinder. Under such nonideal conditions, the preload can decrease to less than 200 N even though the nominal torque of 10 N cm is still applied during tightening of the joint.[58] The explanation for this is that the surface imperfections increase the value of k in equation 10, and as k increases, the preload (F) decreases for the same tightening torque (T). This is significant because it means that a nonideal joint will tend to open at forces lower than the ideal value of 300 N—eg, at 150 to 200 N. This can be a serious clinical problem because tensile forces of more than 150 N can readily occur on implants in the more anterior locations, for example, in the case of a prosthesis with a large cantilever, as discussed earlier in this chapter. Therefore, clinical cases will be predisposed toward screw loosening if non-ideal conditions exist in the screw joint. This may be part of the reason for screw loosening as reported clinically.[59]

Implant loading as a result of misfit of a framework

Most frameworks for full-arch prostheses are made using impressions, stone models, and lost-wax casting technology whose accuracy depends on the skill of the operator and the laboratory. Despite every effort at precision, and despite newer methods of fabricating prostheses such as using computer-aided manufacturing, it is nevertheless possible for the final framework to have dimensional inaccuracies relative to the interface relationships between the framework's fit surface and the actual positions of implant abutments in the oral cavity. *Misfit* is the catch-all term that refers to this mismatch between the prosthesis and the true abutment locations. Assuming that the misfit is not too severe, a given framework may appear to fit well, or *passively*—at least as judged by visual inspection and certain ad hoc physical tests (eg, the Sheffield test[60]). In cases of severe misfit, the clinical concern is that problems may arise down the road with either the implant hardware, the teeth, the framework, or the bone-implant interface. In any case, the origin of the concern is biomechanical and involves screw joint mechanics, as explained below.

The origin of misfit-induced implant loading can be visualized by a free-body diagram of a framework for five abutments

(Fig 6-16). For purposes of discussion, suppose five implant abutments are arranged in a straight line. Assume that during a try-in of the prosthesis, four of the five interfaces match perfectly. However, also suppose that with one of the five abutments, a small gap exists (as a result of manufacturing errors) between the gold cylinder and the abutment. As a result, there is a misfit at that one location, but there is a "passive fit" for the other four abutments. Next, when the four gold screws are torqued down onto the four well-fitting abutments, the ideal preload of about 300 N ought to develop in each joint, and at the end of the torque-down process there should not be any loading of the implants in the distribution; the only "loading" that should exist is the internal preload within each screw joint. However, suppose we now take the last step and start tightening the gold screw at the one abutment where the gap exists. (We're assuming the gap is small enough that the gold screw can reach the internal thread of the abutment screw; Fig 6-16 is exaggerated to make the point.) As we tighten the gold screw up to the target torque of 10 N cm, a tensile force will start to develop in the gold screw, the abutment screw, and the bone-implant interface. However, in the location of the misfit, the tensile preload will also act on the framework, tending to bend it down toward the abutment and diminishing the gap. By Newton's law of action-reaction, this force on the prosthesis is balanced by an equal and opposite force on the implant in the bone, which means that this one implant and its bone-implant interface are now loaded. Now, if the misfit gap were small, it might be possible to close it eventually by continued screw tightening and deformation of the framework, although even after closing the gap, a residual elastic force on

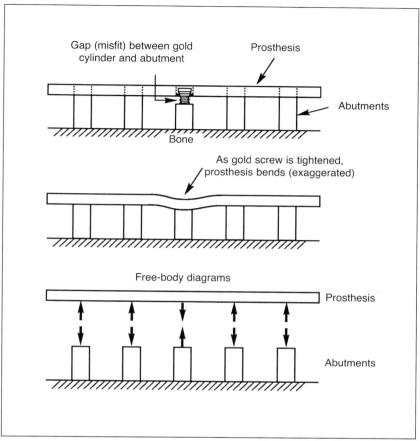

Gap (misfit) between gold cylinder and abutment

Prosthesis

Abutments

Bone

As gold screw is tightened, prosthesis bends (exaggerated)

Free-body diagrams

Prosthesis

Abutments

Fig 6-16 Diagrammatic explanation of how a misfitting framework can cause loads on implant abutments even before any biting force is applied to the prosthesis. (Reprinted from Naert et al[13] with permission.)

the implant parts and the framework could remain until such time as the force in the interfacial bone decayed as a result of stress relaxation in the bone. Along the same lines, if the gap were so large that it did not close by the time the target torque of 10 N cm was reached, again there would be a force on the framework, implant, and interfacial bone at the location of the misfit, which may or may not decay with time. So for both small and large gaps, what happens is that, in a real sense, this force at the misfit location can be considered as an "external" force acting on the framework at that location. In turn, according to the Skalak model, this applied force at the location of the misfit suggests that the other four implants will be loaded by virtue of the misfit at the one location. In other words, the set of five implants ends up being loaded during attachment of the prosthesis, even before any "external" biting forces are applied. The loading due to the misfit is illustrated schematically in the free-body diagram in Fig 6-16.

While the above gives a reasonable initial explanation of the biomechanics of misfit and the way it can cause loading of implants even before masticatory forces are applied, only a few studies have tried to quantify the mechanics or the ultimate clinical consequences of misfit.[11,61] Notably, some studies support the idea that misfit may not be as much of a clinical problem as has sometimes been suggested; for example, some clinical studies have shown that even where there is substantial misfit—eg, on the order of a few hundred microns—major clinical problems with the implant hardware or the bone have not followed.[62] Likewise, animal studies have not revealed major problems in the bone-implant interface in cases of large misfit between the fixed partial denture and implants.[63] Nonetheless, the clinician should strive to achieve as optimal a fit as possible so as to minimize unfavorable loading.

Summary

Although the design of osseointegrated implants and prostheses is not yet a highly exact technology, a quantitative body of knowledge is evolving in the area of implant biomechanics. Biting forces on fixed prostheses are of the same order of magnitude as the forces in the natural dentition. When implants are used to support multi-unit prostheses, biomechanical analyses show that forces on individual implants can be larger than the biting forces on the prosthesis. While this finding may seem surprising, it follows from leverage effects inherent in the geometry of implant placement and the nature of abutment attachment to the prosthesis. The exact force and moment distribution among several implants supporting a prosthesis generally is not measured routinely in clinical cases (nor is the biting force), but estimates of the implant loading can be made using approximate analytic and computer models. These models show, for example, that without cantilevers, the maximum vertical force on any one implant generally will be compressive and less than or equal to the bite force on the prosthesis. At the same time, there can be moments on implants, and these moments depend also on the bite force and exact geometry of the crown. However, when cantilevers exist, the maximum load on the implant nearest the cantilever region can be two to three times the applied bite force, depending on various geometric factors such as cantilever length and interimplant spacing. Naturally, adjustments in the number of implants, cantilever length, and/or interimplant spacing can improve or worsen the situation. There can also be moments on implants when they are freestanding or used in supporting a full-arch prosthesis. Exactly what levels of force and moment are safe versus dangerous to the implant and the bone-implant interface continues to be a major research question, but this subject goes beyond the scope of this chapter. Factors such as (1) implant stiffness in the bone, (2) framework rigidity, and (3) misfit between prosthesis and abutment can influence the manner in which loads are distributed among the abutments. As a general rule, if the goal is to involve as many implants as possible in sharing load support, then all implants should have the same stiffness in the bone and the prostheses ought to be as rigid as possible. While there is still a need for more research on the significance of misfit, it remains prudent to err on the side of caution and plan frameworks that will fit as well as possible to ensure that *(1)* the screw joints can be tightened to produce the optimal preload (clamping force) of, eg, about 300 N between the gold cylinders and the abutments in the Brånemark System; and *(2)* the loading among implants is not worsened by superposition of initial loadings produced by a misfitting prosthesis. These precautions stem from the general idea that one does not want to load the internal parts of the implant screw joint, or the implant itself in the bone, in a manner that is outside the design limits of the system. That being said, it still remains for the field to define more precisely the design limits in view of the expected loadings in vivo.

References

1. Brunski JB, Skalak R. Biomechanical considerations for craniofacial implants. In: Brånemark P-I, Tolman DE (eds). Osseointegration in Craniofacial Reconstruction. Chicago: Quintessence, 1998: 15–36.
2. Brunski JB, Puleo DA, Nanci A. Biomaterials and biomechanics of oral and maxillofacial implants: Current status and future developments. Int J Oral Maxillofac Implants 2000;15:15–46.
3. Brunski JB. In vivo bone response to biomechanical loading at the bone/dental-implant interface. Adv Dent Res 1999;13:99–119.
4. Brånemark P-I, Skalak R. Definition of osseointegration. In: Brånemark P-I, Rydevik BL, Skalak R (eds). Osseointegration in Skeletal Reconstruction and Joint Replacement: Second International Workshop on Osseointegration in Skeletal Reconstruction and Joint Replacement, Rancho Santa Fe, California, October 1994. Chicago: Quintessence, 1997:xi.
5. Brunski JB. Influence of biomechanical factors at the bone-biomaterial interface. In: Davies JE (ed). The Bone-Biomaterial Interface. Toronto: University of Toronto Press, 1991:391–405.
6. Szmukler-Moncler S, Salama H, Reingewirtz Y, Dubruille JH. Timing of loading and effect of micromotion on bone-dental implant interface: Review of experimental literature. J Biomed Mater Res 1998;43:192–203.
7. Brunski JB, Nanci A, Helms JA. Implant stability and the bone-implant interface [editorial]. Appl Osseointegration Res 2000;2:3–5.
8. Soballe K, Brockstedt-Rasmussen H, Hansen ES, Bunger C. Hydroxyapatite coating modifies implant membrane formation. Controlled micromotion studied in dogs. Acta Orthop Scand 1992; 63:128–140.
9. Hoshaw SJ, Brunski JB, Cochran GV. Mechanical loading of Brånemark implants affects interfacial bone modeling and remodeling. Int J Oral Maxillofac Implants 1994;9:345–360.
10. Isidor F. Histological evaluation of peri-implant bone at implants subjected to occlusal overload or plaque accumulation. Clin Oral Implants Res 1997;8:1–9.
11. Duyck J, Ronold HJ, Van Oosterwyck H, Naert I, Vander Sloten J, Ellingsen JE. The influence of static and dynamic loading on marginal bone reactions around osseointegrated implants: An animal experimental study. Clin Oral Implants Res 2001;12:207–218.
12. Hibbeler RC. Engineering Mechanics: Statics, ed 9. Upper Saddle River, NJ: Prentice-Hall, 2001.
13. Brunski JB, Skalak R. Biomechanics of osseointegration and dental prostheses. In: Naert I, v an Steenberghe D, Worthington P (eds). Osseointegration in Oral Rehabilitation. Chicago: Quintessence, 1993:133–156.
14. Rangert B, Gunne J, Sullivan DY. Mechanical aspects of a Brånemark implant connected to a natural tooth: An in vitro study. Int J Oral Maxillofac Implants 1991;6:177–186.
15. Craig RG (ed). Restorative Dental Materials, ed 6. St Louis: Mosby, 1980:60–61.
16. Meng TR, Rugh JD. Biting force on overdenture and conventional denture patients [abstract 716]. J Dent Res 1983;62:249.
17. Ralph WJ. The effects of dental treatment on biting force. J Prosthet Dent 1979;41:143–145.

18. Colaizzi FA, Javid NS, Michael CG, Gibbs CJ. Biting force, EMG, and jaw movements in denture wearers [abstract 1424]. J Dent Res 1984;63:329.

19. Haraldsson T, Karlsson U, Carlsson GE. Bite force and oral function in complete denture wearers. J Oral Rehabil 1979;6:41–48.

20. Carlsson GE, Haraldsson T. Functional response. In Brånemark P-I, Zarb GA, Albrektsson T (eds). Tissue-Integrated Prostheses. Chicago: Quintessence, 1985:155–163.

21. Graf H. Occlusal forces during function. In: Rowe NH (ed). Occlusion: Research on Form and Function. Ann Arbor: University of Michigan, 1975: 90–111.

22. Harrison A, Lewis TT. The development of an abrasion testing machine. J Biomed Mater Res 1975;9:341–353.

23. Ahlgren J. Mechanism of mastication. Acta Odontol Scand 1966;24(suppl 44):100–104.

24. Carlsson GE. Bite force and chewing efficiency. Front Oral Physiol 1974;1:265–292.

25. Glantz P-O, Rangert B, Svensson A, et al. On clinical loading of osseointegrated implants. A methodological and clinical study. Clin Oral Implants Res 1993;4:99–105.

26. Gunne J, Rangert B, Glantz P-O, Svensson A. Functional loads on freestanding and connected implants in three-unit mandibular prostheses opposing complete dentures: An in vivo study. Int J Oral Maxillofac Implants 1997;12:335–341.

27. Richter EJ. In vivo horizontal bending moments on implants. Int J Oral Maxillofac Implants 1998; 13:232–244.

28. Duyck J, Van Oosterwyck H, Vander Sloten J, De Cooman M, Puers R, Naert I. Magnitude and distribution of occlusal forces on oral implants supporting fixed prostheses: An in vivo study. Clin Oral Implants Res 2000;11:465–475.

29. Duyck J, Van Oosterwyck H, De Cooman M, Puers R, Vander Sloten J, Naert I. Three-dimensional force measurements on oral implants: A methodological study. J Oral Rehabil 2000;27:744–753.

30. Mailath G, Schmid M, Lill W, Miller J. 3D-Finite-Elemente-Analyse der Biomechanik von rein implanatatgetragenen Extensionbrucken. Z Zahnnarztl Implantol 1991;7:205–211.

31. Mailath-Pokorny G, Solar P. Biomechanics of dental implants. In: Watzek G (ed). Endosseous Implants: Scientific and Clinical Aspects. Chicago: Quintessence, 1996:291–318.

32. Block MS, Kent JN. The Integral Implant System and the science of hydroxylapatite-coated implants. In: Block MS, Kent JN (eds). Endosseous Implants for Maxillofacial Reconstruction. Philadelphia: Saunders, 1995:223–250.

33. Burgess AV, Story BJ, Wagner WR, Trisi P, Pikos MA, Guttenberg SA. Highly crystalline MP-1 hydroxylapatite coating. Part II: In vivo performance on endosseous root implants in dogs. Clin Oral Implants Res 1999;10:257–266.

34. Skalak R. Biomechanical considerations in osseointegrated prostheses. J Prosthet Dent 1983; 49:843–848.

35. Brunski JB. Biomechanical factors affecting the bone-dental implant interface. Clin Mater 1992; 10:153–201.

36. Brunski JB, Skalak R. Biomechanical considerations for osseointegrated fixtures. In: Worthington P, Brånemark P-I (eds). Advanced Osseointegration Surgery: Applications in the Maxillofacial Region. Chicago: Quintessence, 1992:15–39.

37. Brånemark P-I, Svensson B, van Steenberghe D. Ten-year survival rates of fixed prostheses on four or six implants ad modum Brånemark in full edentulism. Clin Oral Implants Res 1995;6:227–231.

38. Brånemark P-I, Engstrand P, Ohrnell LO, et al. Brånemark Novum: A new treatment concept for rehabilitation of the edentulous mandible. Preliminary results from a prospective clinical follow-up study. Clin Implant Dent Relat Res 1999; 1:2–16.

39. Brånemark P-I. Introduction to the Brånemark Novum concept. In: Brånemark P-I (ed). The Brånemark Novum Protocol for Same-Day Teeth: A Global Perspective. Berlin: Quintessenz, 2001: 9–30.

40. Vasconcelos LW, Franischone CE. São Paulo case report. In: Brånemark PI (ed). The Brånemark Novum Protocol for Same-Day Teeth: A Global Perspective. Berlin: Quintessenz, 2001:63–77.

41. Krekmanov L, Kahn M, Rangert B, Lindstrom LH. Tilting of posterior mandibular and maxillary implants for improved prosthesis support. Int J Oral Maxillofac Implants 2000;15:405–414.

42. Clelland NL, Gilat A, McGlumphy EA, Brantley WA. A photoelastic and strain gauge analysis of angled abutments for an implant system. Int J Oral Maxillofac Implants 1993;8:541–548.

43. Hoshaw SJ, Brunski JB. Mechanical testing of dental implants with and without "intramobile elements" [abstract 1612]. J Dent Res 1988;67:314.

44. Brunski JB, Schock RB. Mechanical behavior of a fibrous tissue interface of an endosseous dental implant. In: Transactions of the 5th Annual Meeting of the Society for Biomaterials. Mt Laurel, NJ: Society of Biomaterials, 1979:41.

45. Weinstein AM, Klawitter JJ, Cook SD. Implant-bone characteristics of bioglass dental implants. J Biomed Mater Res 1980;14:23–29.

46. Schulte W. The intraosseous Al_2O_3 (Frialit) Tuebingen implant. Developmental status after eight years (I). Quintessence Int 1984;15:1–39.

47. Richter E-J, Orschall B, Jovanovich SA. Dental implant abutment resembling the two-phase tooth mobility. J Biomech 1990;23:297–306.

48. Picton DCA. Vertical movement of teeth during biting. Arch Oral Biol 1963;8:109–118.

49. Pesun IJ. Intrusion of teeth in the combination implant-to-natural-tooth fixed partial denture: A review of the theories. J Prosthodont 1997;6:268–277.

50. Naert IE, Duyck JAJ, Hosny MMF, van Steenberghe D. Freestanding and tooth-implant connected prostheses in the treatment of partially edentulous patients. Clin Oral Implants Res 2001;12:237–244.

51. Skalak R, Brunski JB, Mendelson M. A method for calculating the distribution of vertical forces among variable-stiffness abutments supporting a dental prosthesis. In: Langrana NA, Friedman MH, Grood ES (eds). BED. Vol 24: 1993 Bioengineering Conference, held at Breckenridge, Colorado, June 25–29, 1993. New York: American Society of Mechanical Engineers, 1993:347–350.

52. Brunski JB. Biomechanics of dental implants. In: Block M, Kent J (eds). Endosseous Implants for Maxillofacial Reconstruction. Philadelphia: Saunders, 1995:22–39.

53. Brunski JB, Hurley E. Implant-supported partial prostheses: Biomechanical analyses of failed cases. In: Hochmuth RM, Langrana NA, Hefzy MS (eds). BED. Vol 29: 1995 Bioengineering Conference. New York: American Society of Mechanical Engineeers, 1995:447–448.

54. Morgan J, James DF. Force and bending moment distribution among osseointegrated dental implants. J Biomech 1995;28:1103–1109.

55. Elias JJ, Brunski JB. Finite element analysis of load distribution among dental implants. In: Vanderby R Jr (ed). BED. Vol 20: 1991 Advances in Bioengineering. New York: American Society of Mechanical Engineers, 1991:155–158.

56. Brooke-Smith M. The Study of Fatigue Life of Small Gold Locating Screw Used in Osseointegrated Implant Technique [thesis]. Sheffield, UK: University of Sheffield, 1988.

57. Patterson EA, Johns RB. Theoretical analysis of the fatigue life of fixture screws in osseointegrated dental implants. Int J Oral Maxillofac Implants 1992;7:26–34.

58. Carr AB, Brunski JB, Hurley E. Effects of fabrication, finishing, and polishing procedures on preload in prostheses using conventional "gold" and plastic cylinders. Int J Oral Maxillofac Implants 1996;11:589–598.

59. Kallus T, Bessing C. Loose gold screws frequently occur in full-arch fixed prostheses supported by osseointegrated implants after 5 years. Int J Oral Maxillofac Implants 1994;9:169–178.

60. White GE. Osseointegrated Dental Technology. Chicago: Quintessence, 1993.

61. Smedberg JI, Nilner K, Rangert B, Svensson SA, Glantz SA. On the influence of superstructure connection on implant preload: A methodological and clinical study. Clin Oral Implants Res 1996;7:55–63.

62. Jemt T, Book K. Prosthesis misfit and marginal bone loss in edentulous implant patients. Int J Oral Maxillofac Implants 1996;11:620–625.

63. Carr AB, Gerard DA, Larsen E. The response in bone of primates around unloaded dental implants supporting prostheses with different levels of fit. J Prosthet Dent 1996;76:500–509.

chapter 7

Prosthodontic Aspects of Dental Implants

Jeffrey E. Rubenstein, DMD, MS
Brien R. Lang, DDS, MS

Implant prosthodontics has become a widely used treatment option for the replacement of a single missing tooth and rehabilitation of partial and complete edentulism. The prosthodontic phase of implant therapy requires a high degree of skill, attention to detail, and consistency in the management of each patient. All phases of treatment, from the initial consultation to the completion of the definitive prosthesis, must be accompanied by a commitment to long-term follow-up care and maintenance. Today, a large number of implant systems are available for the clinician to use in patient therapy. It is critical that clinicians understand the principles and concepts that support the system(s) selected to be used with their patients and that they continue to expand their experience in implant treatment by using the system(s). Effectiveness in meeting the treatment needs of patients comes with experience and a commitment to continuing education in implant therapy. Equally important are the maintenance of efficacy and the safety of implant ther-

apy on a patient-by-patient basis to further amplify the treatment benefits and quality of life provided by this type of restorative and prosthetic care.

Treatment Planning

Implant therapy has evolved into a variety of treatment options based on the needs of the patient and the competency of the health care provider. A general dentist can manage solely the placement of the implant(s) and the complete prosthetic rehabilitation in some situations. Other situations may require the skills of a periodontist or an oral and maxillofacial surgeon for implant site preparation and placement, with the prosthetic rehabilitation being completed by either a general dentist or a prosthodontist. The decision as to the treatment option selected rests with the dentist initially contacted by the patient.

The information obtained during the patient consultation appointment and the assessment of this information should identify the role of the initially contacted health care provider in the treatment rendered to the patient. Whether the consulted clinician decides to provide all of the implant therapy or part of the treatment with a referral to others, using the team approach, the following procedures are essential to treatment success.

Presurgical consultation and diagnostic workup

A well-organized and well-performed data-gathering process is essential for the successful outcome of anticipated treatment. Data gathered before treatment is used to select the appropriate implants, determine the surgical protocols, and define the nature of the prosthodontic therapy. The data-gathering process should include a consultation with all individuals who will be providing the care if a team approach has been selected. In so doing, the treatment team can mutually assess treatment options and determine, with the patient, the treatment plan.

Prior to implant placement, necessary diagnostic data include panoramic, occlusal, and lateral cephalometric radiographs where indicated; a periapical radiographic series (full-mouth) for the dentate patient; and articulated diagnostic casts. A complete medical and dental history needs to be recorded to determine if contraindications are present that would limit implant placement and success. Implant placement is usually performed under intravenous sedation. However, if the surgical placement of implants is to be done under general anesthesia, then appropriate laboratory blood tests and a chest radiograph are required. For more complex implant therapy, radiographic scans of the jaws likely are needed to permit the assessment of specific implant sites.

Diagnostic mounting

A diagnostic mounting and articulation of the dental casts is critical for presurgical planning, whether a single-tooth, partially edentulous, or complete-arch treatment is planned. A significant amount of information can be obtained from the articulated casts, including assessment of the axial inclinations of teeth, arch form, and interdental/interarch spatial relationships. The articulated casts can be used to perform diagnostic waxups, construct surgical and radiographic stents, and create provisional restorations. Each treatment plan has its own set of requirements and patient needs that must be met prior to surgical placement of the implant(s). The articulated casts assist the clinician and/or treatment team in meeting these requirements and needs.

For single-tooth applications, the diagnostic cast can be used to transfer the bone-mapping data to the cast in determining the adequacy of bone volume for implant placement. The cast can also be used to create a surgical guide for orienting/indexing the implant at surgical placement. The fabrication of a provisional restoration can be made on the articulated cast. The fixed provisional restoration will assist in contouring the soft tissues around the implant site and in creating optimal soft tissue response during the healing phase of treatment. Finally, the cast(s) used for the diagnostic mounting can be used for fabrication of the custom impression tray(s) to be used for making of the final impression(s).

Articulated diagnostic casts are also beneficial when developing a partially edentulous implant treatment plan. The assessment of occlusal relationships and interarch/interdental space is performed using the diagnostic mounting. A diagnostic setup of waxed or denture teeth set in the space to be restored can be used to fabricate a surgical and/or radiographic stent. These preoperative procedures are critical for obtaining ideal implant placement. Presurgical planning provides the clinician responsible for implant placement with a three-dimensional blueprint (surgical guide) that will aid in the successful placement/orientation of the implants within the available bone.

The plan for a completely edentulous patient, whether for a fixed or removable denture, certainly requires no less attention to detail than that for a single-tooth or partially edentulous patient. Articulated diagnostic casts are essential to assess jaw relationships and arch form. It is recommended that the patient's existing dentures not be used to develop the diagnostic mounting or for provisional treatment. Often, the teeth are worn, the occlusion is faulty, or the esthetics are not pleasing. Rather, it is recommended that a set of trial dentures be fabricated to reestablish the vertical dimension of occlusion and the correct centric jaw relation position and to achieve an esthetic result that the clinician and the patient both agree is acceptable. In so doing, the clinician demonstrates control of the treatment to the patient and a dedication to developing a functionally and cosmetically acceptable result right from the start of therapy. Fabrication of new maxillary and mandibular provisional dentures prior to implant placement is the treatment of choice for the patient receiving a full-arch implant-supported prosthesis. In

so doing, the patient can wear the provisional dentures for a week to 10 days prior to the surgery appointment, with any needed adjustment performed prior to implant placement. During the 3 to 4 months of healing following implant placement, the provisional dentures will provide the patient with some degree of comfort, function, and esthetics. At the time of implant uncovering, the denture can be adjusted and/or relined with soft denture liner and worn by the patient until the completion of definitive treatment. This will give the patient an opportunity to become familiar with the support and increased retention provided by the fit of the denture over the abutments and provide feedback as to how the patient is acclimatizing to the converted dentures. This information will be useful when designing the definitive prosthesis. Information on arch form, access for hygiene, speech, and expectations for retention from this initial experience are extremely helpful to the clinician as the definitive therapy is developed and completed.

In more complex cases, the treatment denture can be "converted" into a fixed/detachable provisional by indexing temporary cylinders at each abutment site. This "conversion prosthesis" can offer the patient a prototype for the planned definitive implant-supported prosthesis.

Fabrication of dental casts and mounting them onto a dental articulator will provide a great deal of information about the existing oral conditions of the patient that may not be apparent during the clinical examination. The diagnostic mounting offers the opportunity for the clinician and/or treatment team to design optimal occlusal contacts and determine the need for additional restorative care. Initial selection of the implant design for a patient can be made from the diagnostic mounting. Once the implant has been selected, the choice of surgical approach can be considered.

The use of a diagnostic mounting is invaluable in projecting the goals of treatment, regardless of whether a single implant or a number of implants are to be placed. During treatment planning, mounted casts are essential for diagnosis and the fabrication of implant positioning devices. Without an adequate presurgical workup and the preparation of surgical positioning devices or guides, implant placement may be less than ideal for prosthetic reconstruction. Acrylic templates are easy to fabricate and can make surgical procedures much more effective. A number of techniques are published elsewhere for making guides or stents.[1]

Choosing an implant design

A variety of implant designs have evolved over the years. These designs can be categorized as subperiosteal, transosseous, and endosseous implants. (More discussion regarding these different designs can be found in chapter 1.) This chapter is focused entirely on the restoration of endosseous implant systems, which are currently the most commonly used.

Implant

Generally, endosseous implants consist of an intraosseous component that is surgically placed in the patient's maxilla or mandible. (The protocol for implant placement surgery is described in chapter 4.) Today, it is possible to place implants where native bone is inadequate for implant placement. This is accomplished via various grafting procedures with autogenous bone (eg, iliac crest grafts), alloplastic materials such as hydroxyapatite, and various allo-geneic bone substitutes. Resorbable or nonresorbable membranes are sometimes used in conjunction with grafting for implant site development. The maxillary sinuses (grafted) and the pterygoid region also offer opportunities for placement of implants. Distraction osteogenesis is the latest technique in implant site development, offering an alternative to grafting. The original surgical protocol for implant placement mandated a healing period to allow for osseointegration. In such cases, the implant had a cover screw to protect the internal threading of the implant while it remained submerged beneath the soft tissue. Recently, immediate placement of implants (ie, at the time of tooth extraction) coupled with immediate loading of single- and/or multiple-unit restoration(s) on implant(s) has become another practiced protocol. Alternatively, miniature transitional implants have been used by some clinicians to provide patients with immediate implant-supported (provisional) prostheses during the healing phase of conventional implant therapy. Therefore, the complexity of establishing a treatment plan that includes implant therapy has a much broader scope and requires consideration of the variety of options now available.

Various types of implant surface preparations and/or coatings, eg, acid-etched, sand- or grit-blasted, titanium plasma-sprayed, and hydroxyapatite-coated, have been used in endosseous implant fabrication to enhance their biocompatibility and improve the bone-to-implant interface. Implant collars with either a polished surface or continuous threads up to the top of the implant have recently been introduced as a means to enhance the bone interface. Other proprietary surface characterizations have been introduced for some implant

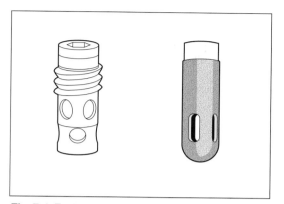

Fig 7-1 Endosseous implants designed as cylinders.

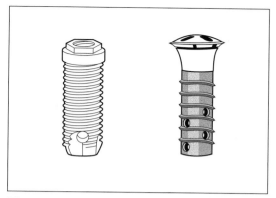

Fig 7-2 Endosseous implants designed as screws.

systems that are claimed to enhance osseointegration.

Implant designs are varied but generally conform to the shape of a natural tooth root. Some implants are designed as cylinders (Fig 7-1). Other implant forms are threaded screws in either a straight or tapered design (Fig 7-2). The endosseous implant is machined from commercially pure titanium or a titanium alloy and is cleaned, sterilized, and packaged in a sterile container ready for use.

The top surface of most early implants was designed with an external-hexagon coupling mechanism.[1] This design permitted engagement of a torque transfer-coupling device (fixture mount) during surgery that assisted in the threading of the implant into bone (Fig 7-3). The hexagon design also served as an indexing mechanism between the implant and the abutment component that brought the implant complex into the oral environment at stage 2 surgery. By the mid 1990s, the number of different implant systems using the external hexagon concept numbered 25.[2,3] Today, the clinician is overwhelmed with more than 90 root-form implants that are available in a variety of diameters, lengths, surfaces, platforms, interfaces, and body designs.[3] Virtually every implant company manufactures a hex-top interface, a proprietary interface, or both. The implants are produced in narrow-, regular-, and wide-diameter bodies with machined, textured, or coated surfaces. A number of implant lengths are also available. In the wide-diameter implants alone, there are at least 25 different offerings with 15 external-hexagon implants and 10 other abutment-implant interface configurations.[3] Recently, implant designs have been introduced that replace the external hexagon with an internal-hexagon design. This internal design is claimed to provide a more stable interface between the top of the implant and the components attached to the implant by screws (Fig 7-4).

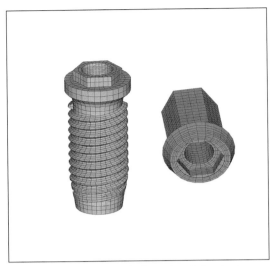

Fig 7-3 The coronal end of most early implants was designed with an external hexagon, which permitted engagement of a coupling device that assisted in the threading of the implant into bone during surgery.

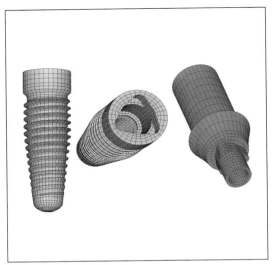

Fig 7-4 Recently, implant designs that replace the external hexagon with an internal design have been introduced. This internal design is claimed to provide a more stable interface between the top of the implant and the components attached to the implant by screws.

Implant abutment

Implant abutments take various forms, which differ in how they receive the prosthetic reconstruction. In most situations, the abutment is joined to the implant by a screw (abutment screw), thus creating a screw joint. The dental prosthesis is placed onto the abutment and fixed using a second screw called the *prosthetic retaining screw*. This second screw is threaded into a screw bore located within the abutment screw. In this screw-within-a-screw design, two screw joints of equal importance are contained within the implant restoration (Figs 7-5 and 7-6). Some systems use a design by which the abutment is attached to the implant by a screw and the dental prosthesis is cemented onto the abutment. However, this latter as-sembly makes monitoring stability of the screw joint impossible without removal of the prosthesis. Such procedures usually require cutting the prosthesis.

Most dental implant research from 1988 to 1994 focused on the success or failure of the bone-to-implant interface with encouraging data on the survival and success of osseointegration.[4–9] However, prosthetic screw loosening and/or fracture, instability of the joint between the implant and the abutment, and fractures of abutment screws were quite common occurrences. The reported rates of such complications ranged from 6% to 48% of the implants placed.[10–27] During the early to mid-1990s, it was estimated that more than one quarter of the patients with prostheses sup-

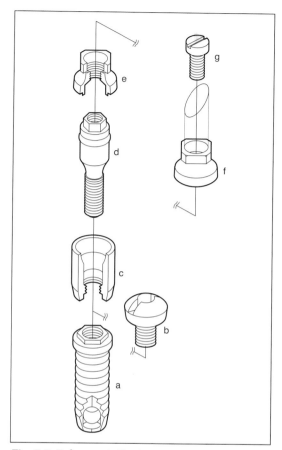

Fig 7-5 Brånemark System components. *(a)* Implant; *(b)* cover screw; *(c)* abutment; *(d)* abutment screw; *(e and f)* cylinder; *(g)* gold screw.

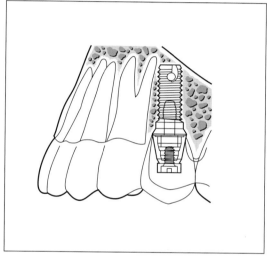

Fig 7-6 The implant core is incorporated into a cast crown, which is attached to the abutment by a gold screw.

ported by dental implants experienced some type of complication during the first 3 to 5 years. Most of these complications were related in some way to instability of screw joints.[26] By the early 1990s, osseointegration of implants into living bone had proven predictable. However, the weakness in implant systems in general appeared to be with the abutment-implant and prosthesis-abutment interfaces. Im-

plant manufacturers, researchers, and clinicians recognized the need to further research those factors that influenced screw joint instability and make whatever improvements were needed to reduce the number of such complications.

Two primary areas of research evolved to address screw joint instability. First, it was hypothesized that new designs at the abutment-implant interface might minimize joint instability. Second, the development of implant screws with greater strength, control of friction, newer materials, and altered surface characterizations was thought to be a way of reducing joint instability.

Abutment-implant interface

The geometry at the abutment-implant connection is one of the primary determinants of joint strength, joint stability, and rotational stability.[3] The long-term clinical data on performance of the abutment-implant connection until the mid-1990s involved implant systems with the external hexagon. This was primarily a result of the dominant use of the Brånemark System (Nobel Biocare, Yorba Linda, CA) worldwide, which uses the external hexagon, and the fact that most new implant systems introduced to the market between 1985 and 1990 were clones of the Brånemark external-hexagon design.

In the mid-1990s, many of the failures and complications that occurred were associated with the abutment–implant screw joint assembly and the prosthetic and restorative procedures.[28–30] It was suggested that the external hexagon and the joint design did not shield the abutment screw from external stress.[3] The screws were subjected to lateral bending loads, tipping, and slipping, which could result in joint opening, joint instability, and screw loosening.[30–35]

At the present time, abutment-implant interface connections are generally described as *internal* or *external* (Figs 7-7 and 7-8). The external joint has the hexagon extending above the bearing surface of the implant. The internal joint assemblies are primarily deep internal joints that often incorporate a rotational resistance and indexing feature. In these designs, the screw theoretically takes

little or no load and the connector provides intimate contact with the implant walls, thereby resisting micromovement. However, data to support their effectiveness have not yet appeared in the literature.

Implant abutments can be subdivided into broad categories, eg, healing, anatomic versus nonanatomic, transmucosal, implant level, emergence profile, angulated, preparable, gold, titanium, ceramic (AlO_2), zirconia, castable (from plastic patterns such as UCLA versus machined metal collars at the implant level with plastic sleeves for developing a wax pattern for casting) and, more recently, computer-designed and -milled components of titanium and ceramic. Just as abutment designs have changed, so have the materials used in abutment manufacturing. Abutments are available in gold alloys, titanium, titanium alloy, aluminum oxide, and zirconium oxide ceramics. This wide array of abutment choices can be overwhelming at first, but their selection and use can be categorized and aligned with various types of treatment, ie, edentulous, partially edentulous, or single-tooth implant restorations.

For the edentulous mandible, the majority of full-arch implant-supported prostheses are fabricated on standard transmucosal abutments. This is the abutment of choice, primarily because it affords ease of maintenance by the patient once the screw-retained restoration is placed. The clinician also has less difficulty in some respects developing the restoration during the impression and fitting phases, since it is easy to access a base foundation that is above tissue level. If the treatment plan calls for having the restoration emanate through the soft tissues, eg, in the case of maxillary treatment, especially in the esthetic zone, then consideration for using implant-level abut-

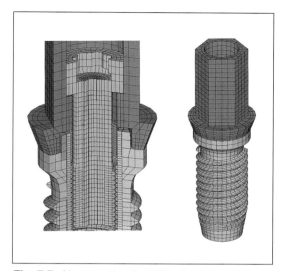

Fig 7-7 Abutment-implant interface connections are generally described as internal or external. The external joint has the hexagon extending above the bearing surface of the implant.

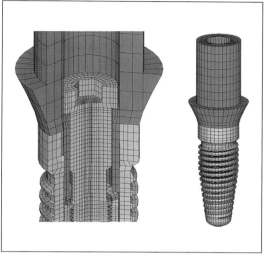

Fig 7-8 Internal joint assemblies are primarily deep internal joints that often incorporate a rotational resistance and indexing feature.

ments or emergence-profile abutments is generally the treatment of choice. Of necessity, sealing the interface of the restoration to the inter- and peri-abutment soft tissues affords more effective management of speech and saliva control with a full-arch maxillary implant-supported restoration. This is often unnecessary for mandibular implant-supported prostheses, but occasionally a tissue-level prosthesis (emergence profile) design might need to be considered, eg, when the patient has a significant display of mandibular teeth and a tall anterior ridge, which would reveal the abutments during activities such as speaking and smiling.

Angulated abutments of inclinations from 17 to 35 degrees or more are available from various manufacturers. These are used to redirect the screw access holes for screw-retained implant restorations from the facial or buccal to the occlusal, lingual, or palatal regions of the restoration or establish an appropriate path of insertion for cemented restorations. Generally speaking, angulated abutments are used to correct the unfavorable axial inclination of an implant resulting from poor placement or less-than-ideal bony anatomy into which the implant is placed.

For partially edentulous implant restorations, a variety of choices exist and can be subdivided into screw-retained or cemented restorations. Multi-unit implant restorations, generally speaking, are best designed as splinted rather than individual units. Thus, it is necessary to have a path of insertion compatible with placement of the restoration.

Screw-retained restorations in nonesthetic areas of the oral cavity are best treated with transmucosal standard abutments, in similar fashion to the full-arch implant-supported prosthesis. Alternatively, emergence-profile abutments or implant-level abutments can be considered for the prosthesis interface.

If a cemented restoration is the treatment of choice, cast, implant-level, preparable, computer-aided design/machining (CAD/CAM) can be employed to achieve a parallel path of insertion for multi-unit restorations. Cements dedicated for a metal-to-metal interface have not yet been developed. As a result, some clinicians elect to permanently cement implant restorations with zinc phosphate, glass-ionomer, or resin dental cements. Others elect to use "soft" cements, such as zinc oxide and eugenol, to address retrievability. In this regard, both cement approaches can often lead to difficult management relative to nonretentive restorations with "soft" cements and to abutment screw loosening with "hard" cements. Screw-retained restorations offer ease of complication management, but clinicians choosing to cement restorations do so because they do not care for screw access holes in their restorations, citing esthetic compromises and limited control in optimizing occlusal contacts as their primary objections.

Single-tooth restorations can be designed to be either screw-retained or cemented. Screw-retained restorations mandate abutment designs that have nonrotational interfaces with the implant body. Likewise, the coping/crown that is screwed to the abutment must have antirotational design. Cemented restorations can be placed on parallel-sided abutments or tapered abutments. Tapered abutments can be prepared and fabricated from gold, titanium, titanium alloy, ceramic, or most recently zirconia. Further, abutments for single-tooth cemented implant restorations can be fabricated by CAD/CAM by milling titanium, ceramic materials, or zirconia.

Although significant improvements appear to have been made in the design of the abutment-implant interface, it must be recognized that the external-hexagon design is still the dominant abutment-implant connector for most implant systems. However, even the external hexagon has undergone changes since its initial introduction in the 1980s. Increases in the height of the hexagon, modifications to the flat-to-flat hexagon widths, and changes in the angulation of the load-bearing platforms of this joint configuration have emerged during the past 10 years.[3] The influence of these changes to the external-hexagon design on screw joint stability has not been reported in the literature.

Implant screw

One of the most critical aspects in the replacement of missing teeth with dental implants is the ability of small screws within the implant complex to hold the various implant parts together during loading and stress transfer. These screws are tightened using a screwdriver that delivers a torque to establish an initial stress level within the screw during tightening, which becomes critical to the maintenance of the joint stability between the parts that the screw is clamping together. Owing to the high strain level that the assembled joint experiences every day from occlusal loading forces, this initial stress level, called the *preload*, is of paramount importance. Insufficient tightening of the screw can result in the screw becoming loose rather quickly, and over time this looseness can lead to fracture of the screw and potentially failure of the implant reconstruction.

During the past 10 years, most manufacturers have altered their screw designs in an attempt to improve the performance of the

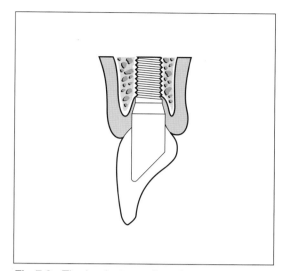

Fig 7-9a The implant core is a dense sintered aluminum oxide that is combined with a veneer porcelain to create the crown restoration.

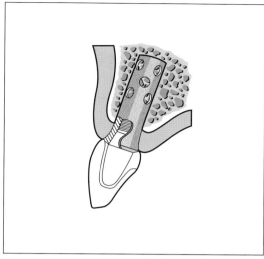

Fig 7-9b The abutment can be custom designed by shaping a titanium blank to the desired form and configuration using dental burs. The crown is then created in a metal-ceramic or an all-ceramic material and cemented onto the abutment.

abutment/implant joint. The focus has been on lowering the loss of input torque to friction, thereby producing a higher preload, which decreases joint instability. An increase in screw stem length to obtain more elongation during tightening and a shortening of thread lengths to reduce friction were among the changes. Changes have also been made in the materials used to fabricate implant screws. Frictional resistance during sliding contact and subsequent wear between the threads in the implant screw bore and the threads of the screw can alter the preload characteristics.[31] Gold alloy screws have been fabricated that can reach preloads of more than 890 N, or approximately 75% of their yield strength. A preload of 75% of the yield strength of an implant screw has been suggested as an optimum preload.[31,36] In an effort to reduce frictional resistance even more, dry lubricant coatings

have been applied to abutment screws. An increase in preload of 24% has been reported by the manufacturer for a gold-coated screw.[3] Teflon-coated screws are also claimed to reduced the frictional coefficient as well. Although these surface coatings may hold promise in influencing joint stability, their effectiveness has yet to be fully documented through independent research and clinical trials.

Abutment fabrication

Most implant abutments are machined in titanium or a titanium alloy to a specific proprietary design for a given implant system. However, some abutments are produced in various ceramic materials; namely, alumina and zirconia oxides. These abutments offer optimal esthetics when combined with an outer layer of porcelain (Figs 7-9a and 7-9b). In still other situations, the abutment is cus-

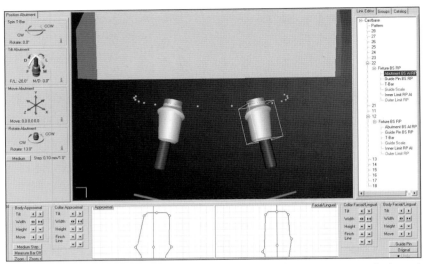

Fig 7-10 CAD/CAM techniques are available to assist in the custom design of single-unit abutments. These methods are used to create abutments that attach directly to the implant and can be created in either metal or ceramic materials.

tom designed by shaping a titanium blank using dental burs in the dental laboratory to the desired form and configuration.

The introduction of CAD/CAM has resulted in a number of approaches to the custom design of abutments to meet alignment, size, and other requirements (Fig 7-10). These CAD/CAM-produced abutments can be manufactured in titanium, as well as the ceramic oxide materials. Adding the veneering porcelain directly onto the abutment or fabricating a crown and cementing it onto the abutment in the conventional manner offers an alternative to a screw-retained single-tooth implant restoration.

Dentition-specific planning

Single-tooth implants
Radiographic information is extremely important when replacing a missing single tooth with an implant. Periapical radiographs can provide valuable information about the space available and the inclination of the roots of the adjacent teeth. Other radiographic procedures, such as axial tomographic imaging and DentaScan (General Electric, Fairfield, CT), providing information that assists in planning implant placement are available. DentaScan images provide life-size (1:1) cross-sectional views that can be used to measure available bone volume and plan for implant length(s) and axial inclination(s). Associated software available with DentaScan allows the clinician to simulate implant placement with various implant designs, lengths, and diameters and even bone grafting procedures such as sinus elevation and onlay bone grafting.

The amount of space between the teeth adjacent to the edentulous area is critical to the success of the single-tooth implant.[37] A space that is too wide will not produce the desired esthetic results. A space that is too narrow to accommodate the implant may be widened by orthodontic therapy. If this will not improve the situation, then prosthodontic options other than implants should be considered.

The contour of the ridge in the edentulous site is equally important. If the bone height is inadequate, it will be difficult to achieve the contour profiles between the implant and the supporting bone that are normally present at the junction of a natural tooth with its supporting tissues. Bone grafting and guided tissue regeneration are techniques that can greatly improve bone and soft tissue contours.

The position of the free gingival tissues on the proximal surfaces of the adjacent teeth is also an important consideration in planning the single-tooth implant restoration. The prosthesis should be designed to provide for access so that maintenance of the tissue, especially in the region of the interdental papillae, can be accomplished. In this way, not only will the appropriate contour of the restoration be established, but also the soft tissues will frame the restoration appropriately to achieve a natural-looking result.

To translate the diagnostic information to clinical application, the clinician placing the implant must be provided with a surgical guide that clearly identifies the desired implant location. The surgical guide or stent design can vary, from being site-specific for single-tooth or partially edentulous treatment to guiding the surgeon to a general area for implants in the totally edentulous arch. The greater the esthetic demands of the anticipated restoration, the greater the need for accurate implant placement and axial orientation.

For delayed (ie, two-stage) implant treatment, placement of a provisional restorations following implant placement will depend on the esthetic and functional demands of the patient. In the anterior part of the maxilla, a provisional single-tooth removable or fixed prosthesis can be fabricated easily, placed, and fully adjusted prior to the surgical appointment. If the removable prosthesis needs to be refitted following surgery or during the healing period, it can be adjusted or relined with a soft denture base lining material. Monitoring the provisional prosthesis during the first few days following surgery is essential. Alternatively, a bonded restoration can be used while waiting for osseointegration to take place. This approach to placing a provisional restoration can be accomplished with a variety of materials and techniques, from cast resin-bonded prosthesis designs, to wire-reinforced bonded denture tooth restorations or composite tooth restorations.

Some clinicians are attempting to immediately place provisional restorations at the time of implant placement. They are designed to be left out of occlusion. Inherent risk of disrupting the connection to the bone can result with this approach; therefore, it is not recommended for the uninitiated implant clinician.

Multiple-tooth spans in partially edentulous arches

When more than one tooth is to be restored, the size of the edentulous area and the amount of bone available for implant placement will influence the number of implants to be placed. In partially edentulous situations, two or more implants are the norm (Fig 7-11). The location of the implants is important to prosthesis design. Arranging artificial denture teeth or using

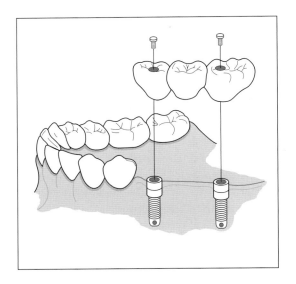

Fig 7-11 The location of implants is important to the design of the multiple-tooth prosthesis. Generally, the implants should be positioned so that the core component can be centered in a tooth within the prosthesis.

wax to develop a full-contour waxup of anticipated replacement teeth for the edentulous area is a common practice used to develop the surgical guide. This approach will also determine how the prosthetic replacement teeth will meet the occlusal demands in rehabilitation. After the diagnostic arrangement of the teeth is completed, the proposed locations for the implants can be decided. Generally, each implant should be positioned so that the abutment component can be centered in each tooth and thereby serve as an anticipated abutment for the prosthesis.

Totally edentulous maxillary and mandibular arches

The diagnostic mounting is often considered unnecessary with the totally edentulous patient. However, failure to use such a mounting may result in a compromise in prosthesis design during treatment that

might have been foreseen and avoided through the study of a diagnostic mounting. Planning via a diagnostic mounting of buccolingual axial inclination, as well as distribution and spacing between implants for the support they will provide either a fixed framework or to retain an implant overdenture for the edentulous arch, is critical. A surgical guide should always be provided for the edentulous arch, as with any other implant treatment. The restorative dentist who delegates implant placement to other clinicians without providing a surgical guide will suffer the consequences if placement is less than optimal. Furthermore, a clinician who does not use a surgical guide for implant placement could be perceived as performing less than the standard of care from a medicolegal standpoint.

A provisional denture is extremely helpful for the edentulous patient who is having implants placed. The sutures are usually removed from the surgical site 7 to 10 days after implant placement, and if adequate healing of the tissues has occurred, a provisional denture can be fitted using a resilient reline material. It is important to monitor the status of the prosthesis, the occlusion, and the integrity of the resilient liner during the healing period between implant placement and abutment connection. Maintenance of tissue health during the healing period between implant placement surgery and uncovering of the implants (stage 2 surgery) is essential.

It is critical when adjusting and relining the provisional denture that the clinician place ample soft reline material between the hard acrylic resin base and the soft tissues. This is true for not only the crest of the ridge but the buccal and lingual borders as well. There should be at least 2.0 mm of soft material to provide a resilient cushion that does not impinge upon the submerged implants. During this time period, the implants are integrating with the surrounding bone, and any excessive force or overload on the implants can cause failure to osseointegrate.

Generally speaking, recall visits every 4 to 6 weeks are adequate for monitoring the health of the tissues and the status of the interim removable prosthesis and resilient liner.

Prosthodontic Procedures Associated with Stage 1 Surgery

If the team approach is selected for implant therapy, it is ideal for the restoring dentist to be present during surgery to assist the surgeon in the decision-making process, even when surgical guides are provided. When it is discovered, for example, that inadequate bone exists at the implant site(s) originally planned, the surgeon and dentist can decide on modifications needed in the implant placement(s) so as not to compromise the definitive prosthesis design.

Another advantage of having the restorative dentist present at stage 1 surgery is that he/she can insert the provisional restorations and make any adjustments that are needed. If the implant site is in the anterior part of the mouth, it is essential that the patient leave the surgery wearing the provisional prosthesis. Many patients are very self-conscious about the esthetics and simply will not go without provisional teeth.

For totally edentulous implant patients, any contact with the surgical site by a provisional denture during the first 7 to 10 days following stage 1 surgery may prove quite uncomfortable and therefore must be delayed. If the provisional denture is worn too early, osseointegration and/or soft tissue healing may be compromised. As soon as it is practical, however, the provisional denture should be placed and maintained for the duration of the healing period. A soft reline material should be used to adapt the denture base to the healing tissue sites (Fig 7-12).

The patient may have questions and concerns and need encouragement while waiting to find out if the implants are indeed integrating with the bone. This waiting period may be very stressful for some patients, and any change in their oral status may cause concern. Replacing the soft lining material several times during the months following stage 1 surgery will do more than just keep the material in good condition; it will show the dentist's concern and provide reassurance for the patient.

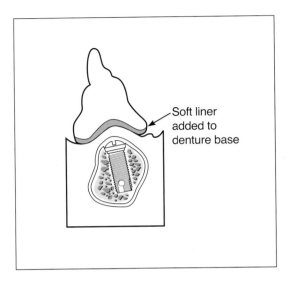

Soft liner
added to
denture base

Fig 7-12 Following stage 1 surgery, a patient's existing denture can be relined with a soft denture base material to serve as a provisional restoration during the 4 to 5 months of postoperative healing.

Prosthodontic Procedures Associated with Stage 2 Surgery

Once the implants are brought into the oral cavity by placement of the abutments during stage 2 surgery, it is important to reemphasize the oral hygiene regimen to the patient so that the tissues around the abutment are maintained properly and kept healthy. For some patients, hygiene will include the use of chemical agents such as chlorhexidine or hydrogen peroxide diluted with water (50/50) or similarly diluted Listerine (Pfizer, New York, NY), in addition to mechanical plaque removal with aids such as floss, yarn proxy brushes, and cotton swabs.

During the 2 weeks of healing following stage 2 surgery where a partially edentulous arch is involved, the provisional restorations may greatly assist in the future prosthesis design by positioning the tissues during healing. Modifications to the tissue surface of the removable provisional prosthesis, eg, relief of some of the acrylic resin base and use of a soft lining material, will permit seating of the prosthesis over the abutments that now extend from the implants. When adequate clearance has been created in the base of the provisional prosthesis to accommodate the abutments, a new application of the soft liner can be placed. This helps to position the healing mucosal tissues around the abutments. This reline procedure where the hard acrylic denture base is of necessity aggressively relieved often weakens the base. To avoid fracture of the provisional restoration, the clinician may reinforce the lingual aspect with wire or fiber; often, this can prevent an emergency repair visit.

Alternatively, a fixed provisional prosthesis can be fabricated to be either screw- or cement-retained by indexing the abutment sites to the provisional restoration with temporary cylinders. Once indexed, the provisional denture prosthesis can be converted (flanges cut back and the prosthesis reinforced with wire embedded in its base on the lingual) to create a prototype of the anticipated fixed restoration. This approach gives the patient an early experience with the anticipated definitive restoration. Further, it provides an opportunity for the patient to learn to develop a protocol for hygiene and maintenance of the fixed restoration, if that is the treatment of choice. If implant overdenture treatment is anticipated, the fixed provisional would not be recommended or possible (generally speaking) relative to the smaller number of implants that are needed to serve as appropriate abutment support, ie, two for an implant overdenture versus four or five for an implant-supported fixed prosthesis.

Once tissues around the abutments begin to show signs of a favorable color response and manipulations of the tissues in the area can be performed without discomfort, the definitive reconstruction procedures can begin. It is important to explain to the patient that following stage 2 surgery, there is no period during which the provisional prosthesis cannot be worn. During the definitive prosthodontic procedures and until completion of the treatment plan, the patient may continue to function with the provisional prosthesis.

Definitive Prosthodontic Treatment

Long-term success with implant therapy can be expected to continue as long as surgical and prosthetic procedures are adjusted to the anatomy, healing potential, hard and soft tissue remodeling capacity, and maintenance capabilities of the patient.[37–39] A tissue-integrated prosthesis can be used to manage a wide range of complex technical and biologic problems involving single-tooth replacement, rehabilitation of the partially edentulous space, and management of the completely edentulous arch. Generally, the prognosis is very favorable for implant therapy when used with these three intraoral conditions. There does not seem to be any advantage to connecting natural teeth and implant abutments in the same fixed implant-supported applications. In fact, a more favorable biomechanical situation is present when the different tooth- and implant-supported prosthetic applications are kept separate. The replacement of lost dentition involving these three oral health conditions can be accomplished with either a screw-retained or a cemented implant restoration.

There are basic prosthodontic treatment protocols for implant therapy involving single-tooth implants, multiple-tooth replacements in partially edentulous jaws, and restoration of the totally edentulous maxilla and mandible. Each treatment protocol has differences or variations in technique for impression making, registration of maxillomandibular jaw relations, implant framework design, and occlusal considerations. Because numerous publications present in great detail each step in the treatment protocols,[37–44] only those aspects of prosthodontic treatment that are uniquely different from conventional prosthodontics in restoring similar tooth loss situations will be discussed here.

Significant progress in the design of implants and related components has been made in the past 10 years. As stated previously, implants are now available in a variety of diameters. The treatment protocols are usually the same regardless of the implant diameter. What is different are the components and instruments that are matched to the diameter of the implant. Beyond these differences, the fabrication of the implant prosthesis and delivery of this health care service are the same.

Single-tooth implants

The principal indication for treatment with the single-tooth implant occurs in anterior and premolar areas where the neighboring natural dentition is intact. In situations where the adjacent teeth have caries and the available space is inadequate for an implant, then conventional prosthodontic treatment using a three-unit fixed prosthesis or a removable partial denture may be the more appropriate therapy.[37] The single-implant restoration is the treatment of choice if the patient's esthetic expectations are realistic. Pronounced bruxism, a short lip, and local vertical resorption of the alveolar process in the edentulous space are factors that would contraindicate the use of the single-tooth implant without further surgery to appropriately develop the site into which the implant can be placed. Perhaps the most compelling reason for single-tooth implant replacement is the required sacrifice of healthy tooth tissue from adjacent intact natural teeth that is necessary with the conventional three-unit fixed prosthesis.

Once the implant is osseointegrated and the clinician is ready to proceed with definitive treatment, several decisions have to be made regarding abutment selection and prosthesis design. When the space available is adequate and the ridge contours are

acceptable, the abutment selection is relatively easy. Decisions about whether to use a transmucosal abutment or a prosthesis design that will originate at the level of the implant are made prior to the start of definitive treatment. However, the achieved surgical positioning of the implant in bone and the soft tissue response during healing will have an impact on these decisions. The transfer of the existing oral conditions to a dental articulator using maxillary and mandibular master casts will provide the clinician with the information needed to make these decisions.

The impression procedure for the single-tooth implant is quite different from that used for conventional prosthodontics for a prepared natural tooth. An implant-level impression is made by first attaching an implant-level impression coping directly to the implant. The impression materials, tray design, and technique will vary depending on the impression coping selected. In this procedure, the impression coping becomes part of the impression and provides the means for transferring the alignment and orientation of the long axis of the implant to the adjacent natural teeth when making the master cast. The impression also records the relationship of the top of the implant to the surrounding soft tissue and free gingival margins.

In most techniques, the impression material is injected around the impression coping, and the impression tray is seated over the coping. The impression coping is removed from the mouth along with the impression when polymerization is completed. An implant replica is connected to the impression coping, and a soft, plasticized acrylic material is placed (via a syringe) around the neck of the coping and over adjacent mucosal margins of the soft tissue

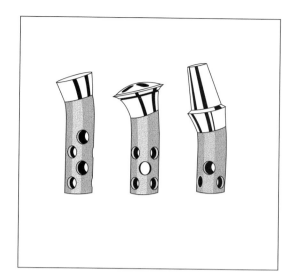

Fig 7-13 Abutments specifically designed to correct for misalignment by adjusting the final angle of the artificial tooth crown.

recorded in the impression. The remainder of the impression is poured in improved dental stone. The master cast created will have the implant replica properly oriented to the adjacent natural teeth and fixed in stone. The soft tissues surrounding the implant will be replicated in a soft material and can be removed from the cast, allowing access to the implant-bearing surface for abutment selection and to facilitate dental laboratory procedures.

When implant therapy was first introduced, the selection of abutments for prosthesis design was limited. As technical innovation has progressed and as our confidence in providing restorations has advanced, patient demands have driven the development of implant abutment choices in the direction of improvement of esthetics. Not only is it important to restore the loss of dentition, but now the aim is to make implant restorations virtually undetectable, especially when replacing missing teeth in the "esthetic zone," ie, the anterior maxilla.

In the single-tooth implant restoration, two basic questions need to be addressed once the casts of the opposing arches have been mounted on the articulator. The initial question is whether a transmucosal abutment will be used or the prosthesis will originate at the level of the implant. Once this decision has been made, the question of whether or not the prosthesis is to be screw retained or cemented can be addressed. If the implant is misaligned, then it will be necessary to address this concern before proceeding to address the two questions. As discussed previously, angulated abutments can be used to correct unfavorable axial inclination of an implant, and are available for either screw-retained or cemented prostheses (Fig 7-13). A CAD/CAM custom abutment can also be designed to compensate for a poorly aligned implant.

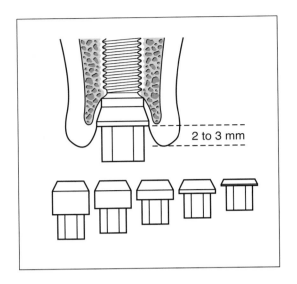

Fig 7-14 Abutment components are available in several lengths to meet the individual needs of different implant sites. The top of the abutment collar should be 2 to 3 mm below the gingival margin.

When alignment and orientation are not of concern and the prosthesis is to originate at the level of the implant, it can be designed to be either screw retained or cemented. In such situations, the prosthesis is usually custom designed to satisfy spatial and dimensional requirements. Additionally, the relationship between the screw-retained or cemented abutment and the implants must have an antirotational design. The single-tooth implant prosthesis design can be developed using preparable abutment blanks in titanium, titanium alloy, or ceramic materials. The prepared substructure can then be finalized using veneering porcelain to complete the tooth form, correct occlusal relationships, and fulfill esthetic requirements. Similarly, the single-tooth prosthetic framework can be fabricated using CAD/CAM technology in titanium, titanium alloy, or ceramic materials.

If the decision has been made to use a transmucosal abutment, a large number of choices are available to the clinician to meet the individual needs of the patient. Abutment components are available in several designs and lengths to accommodate the thickness of the mucosa over the bone (Fig 7-14). The variations in abutment length also provide a means of controlling the placement of the margins of the final implant restoration in relation to the free gingival margins. In the maxillary region, the shorter abutments are most commonly used. With these shorter units, the restoration margins can be placed subgingivally to satisfy most esthetic requirements. Most of these abutment choices also provide prosthetic components that can be cemented onto the abutment or permit screw retention of the final prosthesis to the abutment. The method of incorporating the implant prosthetic components into the final prosthesis is detailed elsewhere.[37–43]

If a cemented restoration is the treatment of choice, abutments that are custom designed can be created for attachment to the implant. The final restoration can then be fabricated using techniques customary for a single crown. The crown is then cemented onto the implant abutment. These abutment forms are created by casting wax patterns specifically created for the implant restoration or developing a preparable abutment; alternatively, a CAD/CAM abutment can be fabricated with an appropriate path of insertion for the final prosthesis.

Cementation of the prosthesis onto the abutment can be achieved with zinc phosphate, resin-reinforced glass-ionomer cement, or resin cements. However, when these cement agents are used, it must be recognized that retrieval of the restoration to check the stability of the fixation screw at the abutment-implant interface usually necessitates the destruction of the prosthesis. Cementation with "soft" cements such as zinc oxide and eugenol affords some degree of retrievability. One drawback of using these soft cement agents is that the prosthesis can become loose. Removal of the prosthesis also can be very difficult when using these soft cements. Screw-retained restorations offer retrievability but come with the drawback of having screw access holes in the area of occlusal contact and an accompanying potential for esthetic compromise.

Multiple-tooth replacements in partially edentulous arches

In general, two or more implants are placed in partially edentulous spaces to support a prosthesis. These multi-unit implant restorations usually involve some form of framework that joins together the implant abutments; thus, it is necessary to have abutments with a path of insertion that is compatible with placement of the restoration. Dental implants can be used in the treatment of multiple-tooth replacements in partially edentulous situations in both the anterior and posterior segments of the maxilla and mandible. Missing central and lateral incisors or a missing premolar and molar in the maxillary arch are good examples of areas in which implants can be used. For these partially edentulous situations, the major decision in prosthesis design is which type of abutment to use. The primary factors influencing this choice are esthetics and oral hygiene access for the patient. If the ability of the patient to practice good oral hygiene is compromised, then the abutment selected must extend through the oral mucosa and provide ample space between the prosthesis base and the soft tissue for the patient to clean the abutments and the undersurface of the prosthesis. If the restoration involves the anterior maxillary arch and the oral hygiene capability of the patient is a concern, then implants are not recommended.

When esthetics is a major concern, the restoration should emanate from the implant through the soft tissues and allow for attachment of the prosthesis to the abutment where the margins of the restoration can be hidden beneath the free gingival tissues surrounding the implants. In so doing, the prosthesis takes on a more natural appearance (Figs 7-15a to 7-15c).

When implants are placed in a partially edentulous ridge, a variety of abutment choices exist to meet both the oral hygiene and esthetic needs of the patient. The available abutment choices accommodate either

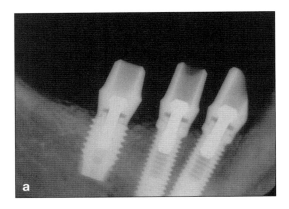

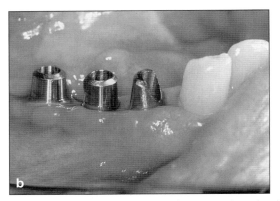

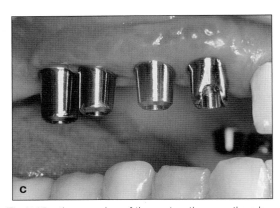

Fig 7-15a When esthetics is the major concern, the abutment should emanate from the implant through the soft tissues. (Courtesy of Dr Michael E. Razzoog, University of Michigan, Ann Arbor, MI.)

Figs 7-15b and 7-15c With the abutment placed as in Fig 7-15a, the margins of the restoration can then be hidden beneath the gingival tissues surrounding the implants. (Courtesy of Dr Michael E. Razzoog.)

screw-retained or cemented restorations. The clinician may elect to defer the final abutment selection until after stage 2 surgery is completed and tissue healing has occurred around the healing abutments. The healing abutments help to guide the tissues in the surgical site in a way that can contribute to the final abutment selection process. They also provide support for the removable provisional prosthesis. If it is unclear which abutment best suits a given situation, the clinician should make an implant-level impression and pour a soft tissue implant analog cast. Once this cast is mounted on the articulator, abutment selection will become much easier.

If a custom or preparable abutment is not the abutment of choice, any number of proprietary abutments can be chosen using the selection kits available for most implant systems. In the anterior maxilla, shorter abutments are most commonly used (Fig 7-16). In the posterior region, longer abutments are the more common choice because the

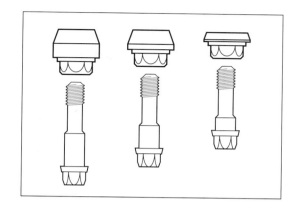

Fig 7-16 Different lengths of titanium collars allow flexibility in the location of the abutment-prosthesis interface.

available vertical space for the definitive prosthesis is usually greater.

The selected abutment can be placed on the master cast and used in the fabrication of the definitive prosthesis. With this approach, the healing abutments and provisional prosthesis can continue to be used by the patient. However, this also means that the abutments must be removed from the master cast and screwed onto the implants during the various try-in and prosthesis construction appointments. When the prosthesis is ready for insertion, the abutments must be thoroughly cleaned and sterilized. Delivery of the final prosthesis involves several steps. First, the abutments are seated onto the implants, and the abutment screws are tightened to the recommended preload. The definitive prosthesis is then positioned onto the abutments and the gold retentive screws are tightened into the abutment screws.

If a custom abutment (preparable or CAD/CAM) or a proprietary antirotational design is selected, then the clinician is faced with a different set of management circumstances. When these abutments are placed onto the implant analogs in the master cast, it must be remembered that 2 to 5 degrees of rotation potential exist at the abutment/implant interface for each implant. This is not a problem during fabrication of the prosthesis if the abutments are never removed from the implant analogs or if no try-ins of the prosthesis are necessary. However, if try-ins are required for fit, esthetics, or other reasons, then there could be major problems. The 2 to 5 degrees of rotation potential can result in differences in the orientation of one abutment to another upon removal and repeated loosening and tightening of the abutments. Should it be necessary to remove the abutments from the implant analogs, then the abutments must be transferred from the master cast to the mouth using an indexing splint. Locking the abutments together using chemically activated acrylic resin is one method for fabrication of the splint prior to removal of the abutments from their implant analogs in the master cast. The splint is kept in position until the abutment is seated onto the implants in the mouth and the abutment screws are tightened. The splint is then removed using burs or other appropriate instruments and the prosthesis try-in is completed. Before the abutments are removed from the mouth, they must again be splinted together to transfer their relationship to one another back onto the master cast.

An alternative to splinting the abutments for transfer to and from the master cast or oral environment is to position and tighten the abutments onto the implants and not remove them throughout the entire prosthesis fabrication process. When these techniques are used, impressions of the abutments should be made in an elastic impression material and dies of the abutment made. These procedures are completed in the dental laboratory. Acrylic resin transfer copings can then be made to fit each abutment die. Clinically, once the abutments have been positioned onto the implants and the abutment screw tightened, the transfer copings are positioned onto the abutments prior to impression making. The copings are picked up in the final impression and the abutment dies are seated into the copings prior to pouring of a soft tissue abutment die master cast. From this point forward, the fabrication of the prosthesis is no different from that for a fixed partial denture. The abutment dies essentially become the tooth preparation dies used in conventional prosthodontics.

This technique avoids the potential for alterations in the orientation of the abutments that can occur when the abutments are continually transferred from the master cast to the oral environment. Additionally, this technique eliminates potential difficulties encountered when attempting to make an impression of the abutments intraorally. For example, it is extremely difficult to record the metal finish line around the abutment when free gingival soft tissues surrounding the implant hide the margin. The use of acrylic resin transfer copings and abutment dies made outside the mouth completely eliminates this problem.

Totally edentulous maxillary and mandibular arches

The rehabilitation of the mandibular edentulous arch with implants involves either a full-arch, fixed, implant-supported restoration or a removable implant-supported overdenture. Primary factors considered during treatment planning include the amount of bone available, the number of implants that the bone will accommodate, and the overall cost of therapy.

Fixed, screw-retained, implant-supported restoration

The mandibular implant prosthesis has traditionally been fabricated on standard transmucosal abutments because most of these edentulous arches demonstrate excessive bone resorption, but not so much that implants would not be supported adequately. These standard abutments allow positioning of the prosthesis above the soft tissue and provide the patient with access for cleaning and oral hygiene.

Impression making of the existing oral conditions and accurate registration of the position of standard or proprietary abutments in the edentulous arch are similar to the techniques used for partially edentulous and single-tooth implant rehabilitation. Various forms of tapered and square copings are used in impression making; however, great care must be exercised in registering the spatial relationships between the abutments. The pouring of the master cast from the final impression differs little from the technique previously described, with the exception that a soft tissue master cast may not be necessary. Regardless of the technique used to create the master cast, its verification for accuracy and replication of the oral conditions are of paramount importance to the success of treatment.

A verification index can be used to ensure that positional and spatial relationships of the implant abutments to each other have been accurately recorded in the impression and transferred to the master cast. Screw-retained impression copings are the component most often used to make a verification index. After the copings have been fitted to their analogs in the master cast, they are united using a chemically activated or light-activated acrylic resin. The copings must fit the abutment-bearing surfaces accurately and passively to ensure a precision fit at their interface during index construction.

The verification index must fit the abutment replicas on the master cast and the abutments in the mouth identically. With the index, it is possible to confirm that the correct spatial relationships of the implant abutments have been recorded and transferred from the mouth to the master cast. The detailed steps in fabrication of the verification index are described in other texts[1,37] and will not be presented here; their importance in implant-supported prosthodontics, however, cannot be overemphasized.

Record bases are necessary in the totally edentulous situation to record and transfer the maxillomandibular relationships from the patient to the articulator. Incorporation of the prosthetic component or temporary cylinder for the abutment selected in the record base will increase stability and provide the retention to ensure accurate registration and transfer. Once the jaw relation records have been obtained, the maxillary and mandibular casts are mounted on the dental articulator at the proper vertical dimension of occlusion.

Once the tooth arrangement has been accomplished, the vertical dimension and centric relation verified, and esthetics approved by the patient, a matrix is fabricated of stone silicone putty or light-cured resin that relates the tooth position to the implant position. This matrix assists the laboratory technician in identifying the available space between the anticipated tooth position and that of the abutment positions to develop and fabricate the framework. If the prosthesis design will incorporate cantilevers extending from the most posterior implant abutments, it is necessary to have a framework that provides adequate strength to the prosthesis base. This framework may be either completely embedded in the prosthesis or form a part of the prosthesis base, to which acrylic resin and replacement teeth are attached (Figs 7-17a to 7-17c).

The cast framework has been the predominant design used to date, but other designs have recently been introduced. These include one-piece machined titanium and carbon-fiber frameworks, both of which are very strong. The carbon-fiber design provides the technician with the opportunity of molding the framework directly onto the implant abutments on the master cast before it is polymerized to the hardened form. Procedures to fabricate such frameworks will be discussed later in this chapter.

If a cast metal framework is selected for the implant therapy, then a wax pattern for the definitive restoration is prepared by incorporating the prosthetic components specific to the abutments into the framework pattern. The pattern design is influ-

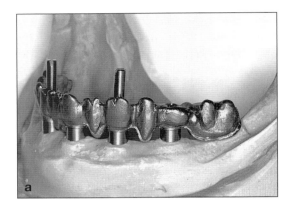

Fig 7-17a In partially or fully edentulous implant therapy, components are incorporated into a wax pattern that is cast in an alloy to form a substructure framework. The framework may take the form of several teeth to which porcelain can be fused, creating the replacement tooth forms.

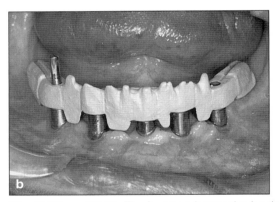

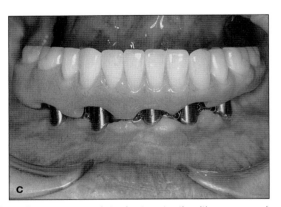

Figs 7-17b and 7-17c The framework may also be designed to accommodate denture teeth with processed acrylic resin. The prosthesis is joined to the implants using gold retention screws.

enced by the materials to be used in the final restoration. The pattern for a porcelain-fused-to-metal restoration is similar to that used for traditional fixed prosthodontics and, as always, the metal casting is evaluated intraorally before the restoration is completed. The implant metal framework must seat completely and passively. Any discrepancy will require the framework to be sectioned, a new relationship secured, and

the framework reunited. When a precise fit is attained, the restoration can be finished by the addition of the desired esthetic material. When porcelain is used to restore function, form, and esthetics, the appropriate supporting surface must be developed in the framework wax pattern. Porcelains selected for this purpose must fuse at temperatures compatible with the metal of the framework.

If composite or acrylic artificial teeth are to be added to the implant framework, a means of retention must be developed, either in the wax pattern or once the framework is completed. The processing of the artificial teeth onto the framework is accomplished in the traditional manner described elsewhere.[1,37]

The occlusal considerations for the mandibular implant prosthesis will depend on the condition of the maxillary arch. If the maxillary arch comprises natural teeth or a combination of natural teeth and fixed partial dentures, then canine-guided or mutually protected schemes are used to release the implant prosthesis from laterally directed forces. The group-function occlusal scheme (multiple working-side contacts in lateral excursions) is equally appropriate, especially for those patients in whom the distribution of forces over several implants is desired. If the opposing arch is a denture, then a lingualized occlusion concept with some degree of lateral occlusal balance is appropriate. This occlusal scheme will more equally distribute the forces to the maxillary denture and its supporting tissues, an important consideration given the greater functional forces that will be experienced as compared to treatment with complete dentures.

For the maxillary full-arch implant prosthesis, the traditional treatment plan usually calls for the restoration to appear as natural teeth emanating from the soft tissues. In this situation, certain proprietary implant abutments are available that permit positioning of the prosthesis in direct contact with the adjacent mucosa surrounding and between the implants. A slight space between the soft tissue and the prosthetic base will permit oral hygiene procedures similar to those used with a fixed partial denture. With these designs, the restoration will appear to be emerging directly from the gingiva. Excellent esthetic results have been obtained using metal frameworks with porcelain teeth. The implant-level prosthesis design can also be used in the mandibular arch when a patient demonstrates a significant display of mandibular teeth and the potential exists for visualization of the transmucosal abutments during activities such as speaking and smiling.

An implant-level impression and soft tissue master cast are required for the maxillary full-arch implant prosthesis if the restoration must appear similar to natural teeth. A record base is again necessary to record and transfer the appropriate maxillomandibular relationships from the patient to the articulator. Once the jaw relation records have been registered, the maxillary and mandibular casts are mounted on the dental articulator at the proper vertical dimension of occlusion, and the prosthesis design is finalized.

A framework that emanates from the implant-bearing surfaces can be designed in wax and acrylic using prefabricated, shaped forms available for the various implant systems. The framework pattern, when completed, can be cast in titanium or some other suitable metal as a one-piece casting or in a segmented solder/assembly approach. CAD/CAM techniques are available that can be used to design and machine a one-piece framework in titanium (Fig 7-18).

Development of the occlusion and the desired esthetics usually involves the addition of ceramic materials to the metal framework. The ceramic material chosen must be compatible with the metal of the framework. When finalized, the prosthesis

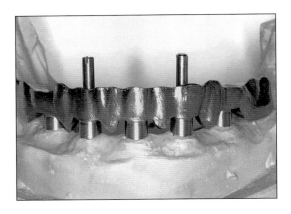

Fig 7-18 A specially designed one-piece machined titanium framework.

is attached to the implants using abutment screws tightened to the appropriate torque.

Fixed, cemented, implant-supported restoration

In some clinical situations, implant treatment of the edentulous arch will use custom abutments. These abutments are either prepared with dental instruments or designed and manufactured using CAD/CAM technology. Implant placement may have resulted in alignment and orientation problems that will not permit the use of a one-piece, screw-retained framework. In such situations, custom abutments can be used to align the abutments and create a path of insertion for the framework. Depending on the amount of alignment correction needed, the framework may be fabricated as one piece or in two to three shorter segments. The full-arch reconstruction thus becomes a series of short-span, implant-supported, fixed partial dentures cemented onto the abutments. In this situation, impressions of the abutments should be made in an elastic impression material, dies poured in stone, and acrylic resin transfer copings fabricated.

Clinically, the abutments are positioned onto the implants and the abutment screws are tightened. The transfer copings are then positioned onto the abutments and picked up in the final impression. The abutment dies are next seated into the copings prior to pouring a soft tissue abutment die master cast. From this point forward, the fabrication of the prosthesis is no different than for a full-arch cemented fixed partial denture. The abutment dies become tooth preparation dies used in fabricating the one-piece or multiple-short-span, implant-supported fixed partial dentures.

Removable implant-supported overdenture

The ideal oral rehabilitation of the totally edentulous arch is a fixed implant-supported prosthesis (Figs 7-19a and 7-19b). Patients who have been provided this service have

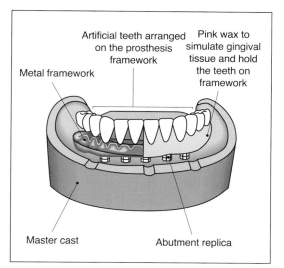

Artificial teeth arranged on the prosthesis framework

Pink wax to simulate gingival tissue and hold the teeth on framework

Metal framework

Master cast

Abutment replica

Fig 7-19a A master cast shows the prosthodontic simulation of a fixed implant-supported prosthesis for a totally edentulous mandible.

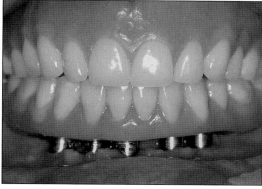

Fig 7-19b Fixed implant-supported mandibular prosthesis opposing a maxillary complete denture.

reported satisfaction with the improved function and comfort. However, this approach is not always possible. Anatomic and functional limitations that preclude the use of a fixed prosthesis are present in some patients. However, the most common reason for selection of an overdenture instead of a fixed prosthesis is one of economics.

If loss of the natural teeth and the alveolar bone associated with their support has created severe anatomic deficiencies, then the treatment of choice is an implant-supported overdenture. If the bone quantity and quality available limit the surgeon to placement of only two or three implants, then an overdenture is also indicated. If four or more implants can be positioned appropriately, and anatomic features are not limiting factors, then a fixed prosthesis is the restoration of choice. Esthetic and phonetic problems are associated with severe resorption and tooth loss. The lost bulk associated with a resorbed alveolus can be restored with an implant-supported overdenture, and esthetic and phonetic problems associated with the loss of these tissues can be avoided. If maintenance of oral hygiene will be compromised by treatment with a fixed prosthesis, then an overdenture is the treatment of choice. Likewise, patients with jaw defects or unusual jaw relationships who would experience adverse biomechanical conditions if restored with a fixed prosthesis should instead receive an implant-supported overdenture.[1,37] In the mandibular arch, treatment with an implant over-

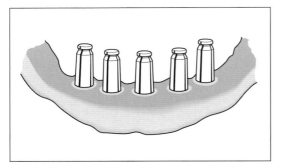

Fig 7-20 Tapered impression copings screwed to the abutments.

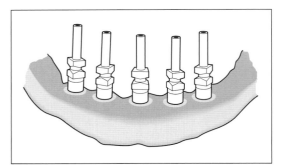

Fig 7-21 Square impression copings are used to make the final impression. These copings are usually joined using a chemically activated acrylic resin, maintaining their spatial relationships during impression making.

denture is rapidly becoming the standard of care. However, this does not mean that an implant prosthesis in the maxillary arch is unnecessary or undesirable. Well-made conventional maxillary complete dentures have resulted in reasonable success rates for edentulous patients. However, the retention achieved with a conventional maxillary denture is not always acceptable to some patients, and implants have been suggested to improve retention for these patients. For patients with excessive resorption of the maxillary ridge or other anatomic considerations that preclude successful denture wearing, the implant-supported prosthesis can be an excellent treatment option.

Impression making of the edentulous arch and accurate registration of the spatial relationships of the abutments are completed using a technique similar to that used for multiple-tooth replacements. The preliminary impression is made with irreversible hydrocolloid with the tapered coping in place on the abutments (Fig 7-20). The copings are removed from the mouth and connected to the abutment analogs. The coping-abutment assemblies are inserted into the impression and a cast is poured in improved stone. For some situations, this cast has been used as the master cast. In other situations, this cast is used to construct a custom impression tray and the making of a second impression to prepare the master cast.

This alternate final impression procedure involves screw-retained impression copings. The design of these copings is such that they become locked into the impression material (Fig 7-21). This impression cannot be removed from the oral cavity unless the retaining screws used to hold the copings in position are loosened and removed from the mouth. Screw removal is facilitated by placement of a window in the top of the impression tray that permits access to the

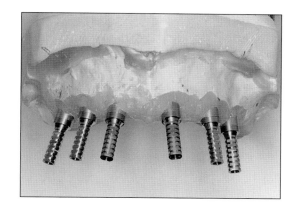

Fig 7-22 Accurate, stable, and retentive record bases are required to record and transfer the appropriate maxillomandibular relationships from the patient to the articulator. Various components can be attached to the transmucosal implant units in preparation for their incorporation within acrylic resin when forming the record base. (Courtesy of Dr Marianella Sierraalta, University of Michigan, Ann Arbor, MI.)

top of the coping retaining screws. After the screws are loosened, the alternate final impression can then be removed intact with the impression copings.

Custom impression trays are made for the final impression procedure using a preliminary cast of the edentulous arch. It is important that the impression record the primary residual ridge and retromolar pads. These anatomic landmarks are important in determining the occlusal plane location in the final restoration for both fixed and removable implant-supported prostheses. The tray for a removable prosthesis is designed for complete border molding, similar to impression making for a conventional denture. In both trays, a relief space is required in the area of the implants to provide for a sufficient thickness of impression material around the impression copings.

For the overdenture implant prosthesis, screw-retained impression copings must be accurately seated on their respective abut-

ments. If only two implants were placed in the edentulous arch, the clinician may or may not choose to lute them together using an acrylic resin material. The final impression is made using any of the number of impression materials available. The master cast is poured in improved dental stone.

A verification index is used to ensure that the positional relationships of the abutments to each other are correctly recorded in the impression and that this relationship has been transferred to the master cast.

Accurate, stable, and retentive record bases are required in the totally edentulous situation to record and transfer the appropriate maxillomandibular relationships from the patient to the articulator. Incorporation of an impression coping, gold cylinder, or a provisional cylinder within the record base will provide the necessary stability and retention when screwed to the abutment and ensure accurate registration and transfer of jaw relationships (Fig 7-22).

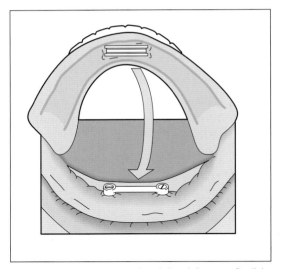

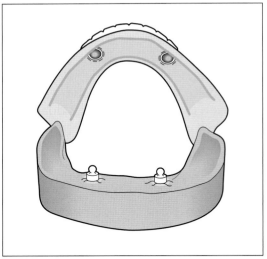

Fig 7-23 Implants can be joined by nonflexible bars, which are used with resilient bar attachments. These implant frameworks provide excellent retention for overdentures.

Fig 7-24 Implants can also be used as single units, with ball attachments to provide overdenture retention. The use of spacers and rubber O-rings allows rotation around the ball, while the support of the posterior mandibular areas restricts tilting.

The design of the record base is similar to the extension and form used in conventional complete denture prosthodontics.

The master casts are mounted on the dental articulator in centric relation. Once the vertical dimension of occlusion and centric relation records are transferred to the articulator, they must be verified by a second interocclusal record. A protrusive record is used to set the condylar elements of the articulator to the degree mechanical equivalents that will simulate the horizontal shape of the patient's condylar eminence, to be used in the arrangement of the replacement teeth on the record base.

Selection and arrangement of the artificial teeth are usually completed before construction of the implant framework, regardless of whether the prosthesis is fixed or an overdenture. There are tooth designs

developed specifically for implant prostheses that maximize control over the direction of the applied forces. Whenever possible, these designs should be used.[10] The principle of lingualized articulation and occlusion has proven very successful in patients with implant-supported restorations. For this arrangement, there are a number of factors that influence the positioning of the artificial teeth in the dental arch. These factors include the incisal guidance and the amount of vertical and horizontal overlap of the maxillary anterior teeth with the mandibular anterior teeth. Minimizing the vertical overlap and maximizing the horizontal overlap within the limitations of an acceptable esthetic result will reduce the occlusal forces at the anterior residual ridge. The positioning of the occlusal surfaces of the mandibular teeth in relation to the corners of the mouth and the retromolar pads in an anteroposterior relationship provides the appropriate occlusal plane for mastication and distribution of the forces from function. The buccolingual placement of the mandibular teeth in relation to the crest of the residual ridge ensures the proper arch arrangement for interdigitation of the mandibular teeth with their maxillary counterparts. Finally, the arrangement of the mandibular teeth with anteroposterior and mediolateral compensating curves ensures that the contacts with the opposing maxillary teeth will be smooth and glide freely during movements of the mandible into lateral positions.

In most situations, the removable implant-supported overdenture treatment plan will involve two implants. The implants may be joined together by a bar (Fig 7-23). The prosthetic components, which precisely fit the implant abutments for the selected implant system, can be incorporated within a cast bar or soldered to a preformed gold bar. The bar is then positioned onto the abutments and rigidly held in place by prosthetic retaining screws. Various clips or other retentive mechanisms that engage the bar unit are incorporated into the denture base.

There are also a number of proprietary systems that involve unique, single-unit, retentive attachments that unite the overdenture directly to the implants (Fig 7-24). Special retentive mechanisms designed for these components are incorporated in the denture base during the processing of the prosthesis. In some situations, an area is developed within the denture base to incorporate soft denture lining material that provides the retentive mechanism for these attachments.

Implant Framework Design and Fabrication

Depending on the treatment plan, ie, single tooth, partially edentulous, or fully edentulous, framework design and fabrication are done using different techniques.

Single-unit framework

Single-tooth restorations can be fabricated with proprietary unit designs that are incorporated within a wax pattern and cast in metal to create the substructure needed for the restoration. A ceramic material of an appropriate shade is then fused to the substructure, creating the form that is needed to satisfy the functional and esthetic needs of the patient. There are also ceramic and titanium proprietary units designed to attach directly to the implant. These units are then prepared for a crown using conventional techniques. If the abutment is made of ceramic material, other porcelains can be fused directly to it to create a restoration with the appropriate contours and esthetics. If the abutment is in metal, porcelain veneer materials are also available for direct fusing to the abutment. These custom abutments can also be designed in a form representing a prepared natural tooth. A single crown restoration can then be fabricated in ceramic material fused to metal and cemented onto the abutment. There are also copy milling and CAD/CAM techniques available for custom designing a single-unit abutment (Figs 7-25a to 7-25e). These methods are used to create abutments that attach directly to the implant and can be created in either metal or ceramic materials.

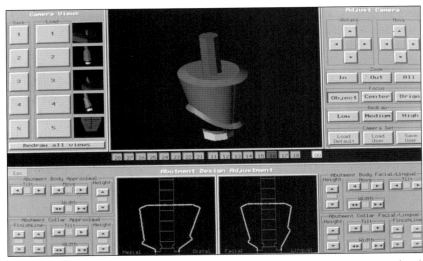

Fig 7-25a The CAD/CAM method can be used to design a single screw-retained titanium abutment. (Courtesy of Dr Michael E. Razzoog.)

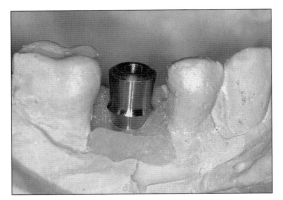

Fig 7-25b The CAD/CAM-produced titanium unit can be designed to emanate directly from the implants.

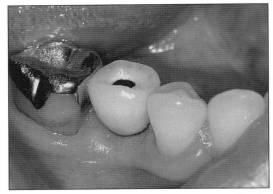

Fig 7-25c Porcelain material can be fused directly to the screw-retained titanium unit.

Multiple-unit, partially edentulous framework

The multiple-unit, partially edentulous framework is created much like the single-unit framework. These frameworks can be fabricated with proprietary abutment units incorporated in a framework pattern that is created in wax or an acrylic resin material. The patterns are then invested in a suitable material and cast in a gold alloy or titanium alloy.

If a custom framework design is required for the prosthesis, then a pattern is created

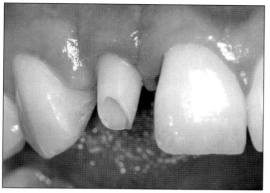

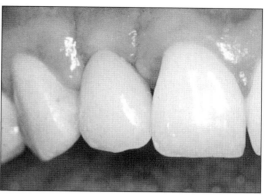

Fig 7-25d The CAD/CAM-fabricated abutment can be created in an all-ceramic material that emanates directly from the implants. (Courtesy of Dr Marianella Sierraalta.)

Fig 7-25e An all-ceramic crown can then be cemented onto the all-ceramic abutment, thereby achieving the best possible esthetic results. (Courtesy of Dr Marianella Sierraalta.)

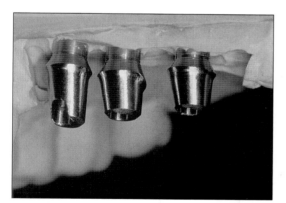

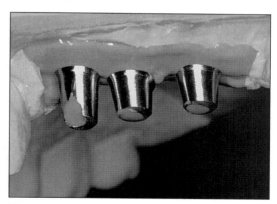

Fig 7-26a The custom abutments generally are designed with the finish line beneath the gingival margin, as determined by measurements made from the implant-bearing surface to the soft tissue margin. The alignment of the CAD/CAM-created abutments can be checked on the master cast. (Courtesy of Dr Matthew Hopfensperger, University of North Carolina, Chapel Hill, NC.)

Fig 7-26b The finish line of the custom abutments is positioned beneath the gingival margin. (Courtesy of Dr Matthew Hopfensperger.)

that emanates from the surface of the implant through the mucosa. In these situations, the interface between the framework and the implants is of a non-hexed design to eliminate potential precision of fit and im- plant alignment problems. The framework can be invested and cast in a suitable metal or designed and machined using CAD/CAM procedures (Figs 7-26a and 7-26b). These custom frameworks are usually manufac-

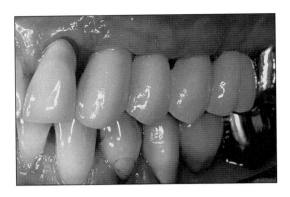

Fig 7-27 The definitive multi-unit, implant-supported fixed partial denture. (Courtesy of Dr Matthew Hopfensperger.)

tured in commercial-grade titanium or a titanium alloy. Frameworks can be designed to allow for the direct addition of a porcelain veneer material, creating the tooth forms and esthetic results required (Fig 7-27). Frameworks can also be designed to receive separate, multi-unit implant prostheses, and all of these designs can be fabricated for either screw- or cement-retained prostheses.

Multiple-unit, fully edentulous framework

Much has been written and researched regarding framework design for the edentulous full-arch restoration. Generally speaking, full-arch implant frameworks are cast using various alloys such as type IV gold, or low-gold-content, silver-palladium alloys. Cast titanium alloy has also been used, but to a lesser degree because of the difficulty in casting titanium and achieving an acceptable precision fit with the implant units.

Multiple-unit, full-arch framework designs can also be machined or copy milled from prepared patterns or using CAD/CAM meth-

ods. These frameworks are manufactured in titanium or titanium alloys. Frameworks can be designed to allow for the desired esthetics. The metal framework can also be designed for incorporation into a denture base of acrylic resin where the occlusion is restored with denture replacement teeth. These frameworks are screw retained either to an abutment or directly to the implant. In certain situations, particularly in the maxillary arch, a multiple-unit framework can be designed that will receive a cemented fixed prosthesis. In these situations, the abutments (designed similar to prepared teeth) are first screwed to the implants, and the prosthesis (similar to a conventional fixed partial denture) is cemented into place.

Recently, a carbon fiber framework has been introduced for edentulous multiple-unit situations. A resin material within a plastic tube that contains the carbon fibers is adapted to proprietary abutments positioned on the master cast. These abutments become part of the carbon fiber framework and will be attached to the implants. When the plastic tube is adapted to the abutments, it is placed in an oven to complete the polymerization process of the resin material. When totally polymerized, the carbon fiber framework is placed on the master cast and incorporated into the denture base, which is formed in wax, and eventually polymerized in acrylic resin during the processing of the prosthesis. The carbon fiber implant framework is very strong and is a cost-effective way of creating a screw-retained, fixed implant prosthesis for the edentulous patient.

Multiple-unit edentulous frameworks can also be designed to receive an overdenture. Overdentures for the mandible can be fabricated by splinting implants with cast or premachined bars of various configurations, eg, round, Dolder, or Hader bars. These bars can then be used to create retention for the prosthesis via clips made from gold alloy or polymers. Splinted designs can incorporate other types of retentive elements, such as resilient attachments, of which there are numerous proprietary designs for the clinician's selection. Space requirements vary from patient to patient, as do implant position and arch form.

For maxillary implant overdentures, conventional wisdom suggests a splinted bar design, preferably with four or more implants. Some patients insist on removal of the palatal coverage that is customary with complete dentures. The splinted framework design with an overdenture does permit the elimination of the palatal portion of the prosthesis for these patients. However, removal of the palatal coverage reduces the support for the prosthesis afforded by the palatal denture base, thereby jeopardizing the implants in patients where bony support is limited. Therefore, it may not be prudent to remove palatal coverage in all patients.

Spark-erosion prostheses or milled bars with electric discharged machined caps are other designs for overlay/removable implant prostheses. A design involving caps on machined/milled bars offers a reinforced beam structure that transmits load evenly to the underlying implants. This may offer a more favorable load distribution when the prosthesis is lacking palatal coverage.

The recently introduced one-piece machined titanium framework offers yet another excellent approach for rehabilitation of the edentulous arch. The pattern design for the implant framework is established after the teeth have been arranged and the clinical try-in completed using the trial base. A silicone putty tooth index, keyed to the master cast, provides the technician with the needed information to fabricate the framework pattern. This index allows determination of the available space between the teeth and the implant cores, where the framework will be formed.

This framework employs a CAD/CAM method that fabricates the framework in one piece in a titanium alloy, exhibiting excellent fit with other implant components. The one-piece custom framework can be designed to emanate directly from the implants. The addition of porcelain veneer material to the framework can then be completed. This framework can also be used in patients who need additional support in the form of a denture base and a prosthesis that emanates directly from the implants. In these situations, elements of the framework must be designed to allow for the addition of denture teeth and the supporting acrylic resin.

If the framework is to be positioned off the tissues, then it is important that at least 2 to 3 mm of space exist between the soft tissues and the undersurface of the implant-supported framework. A space of less than 2 mm makes it difficult for patients to maintain an acceptable level of oral hygiene. The contour of the tissue surface of the framework should be convex to facilitate cleansing, and the faciolingual dimension of the prosthesis must be kept minimal to facilitate access for oral hygiene. All of these design considerations are incorporated into the framework pattern prior to the start of the CAD/CAM machining process for the one-piece framework.

All metal frameworks should be evaluated intraorally, both visually and radiographically, before completion of the restoration. Accurate fit at the prosthodontic interface between the framework and the abutments of the framework and the implants is crucial to the biomechanics of the implant-supported prosthesis. If the elements are misaligned, the magnitude and direction of forces transferred from activities such as chewing may exceed the tolerable limits at the implant-bone interface. A gap between the abutments and the prosthesis could produce uneven force distribution, which could negatively affect the prognosis of the implants. If misalignment is observed, either visually or radiographically, the problem must be corrected before proceeding with any further prosthodontic procedure. In the case of the carbon fiber framework, a proprietary adjustable abutment design is available that can be used to correct for fit concerns.

Research has demonstrated that forces generated by patients with implants during maximum occlusion have approached the forces registered by patients with natural dentitions. In some instances, maximum occlusal forces for implant patients have exceeded those of the dentate patient.[43,44] Therefore, in a totally edentulous implant patient with a full-arch implant-supported prosthesis that opposes an arti-

ficial dentition, it is essential that an occlusal scheme be used that is capable of distributing occlusal forces evenly over the entire opposing arch and equally to each abutment. Bilateral balance and the concept of lingualized articulation are recommended, because the tooth forms associated with this occlusal scheme require less occlusal force to achieve mastication, and there are no deflective occlusal contacts in the various jaw movements.

Posterior implants should maintain occlusal contact in maximum intercuspation. It is recommended that if adequate anterior guidance with the natural dentition exists, the implant-supported restoration should be free of contacts with the opposing dentition during lateral and protrusive jaw movement.

Completion of Restorations

Processing and finishing of implant restorations is somewhat different than for conventional fixed or removable prostheses. Information regarding these techniques can be found in the previously cited implant texts.

References

1. Brånemark P-I. Introduction to osseointegration. In: Brånemark P-I, Zarb GA, Albrektsson T (eds). Tissue-Integrated Prostheses: Osseointegration in Clinical Dentistry. Chicago: Quintessence, 1985: 11–77.
2. English CE. Externally hexed implants, abutments, and transfer devices. A comprehensive overview. Implant Dent 1992;1:274–283.
3. Binon PP. Implants and components: Entering the new millennium. Int J Oral Maxillofac Implants 2000;12:76–91.

4. Cox JF, Zarb GA. The longitudinal clinical efficacy of osseointegrated dental implants: A 3-year report. Int J Oral Maxillofac Implants 1987;2:91–100.

5. Worthington P, Bolender CL, Taylor TD. The Swedish system of osseointegrated implants: Problems and complications encountered during a 4-year trial period. Int J Oral Maxillofac Implants 1987;2:77–84.

6. Engquist B, Bergendal T, Kallus T, Linden U. A retrospective multi-center evaluation of osseointegrated implants supporting overdentures. Int J Oral Maxillofac Implants 1988;3:129–134.

7. Gregory M, Murphy WM, Scott J, Watson CJ, Reeve PE. A clinical study of the Brånemark dental implant system. Br Dent J 1990;168:18–23.

8. Arvidson K, Bystedt H, Frykholm A, von Konow L, Lothigius E. A 3-year clinical study of Astra dental implants in the treatment of edentulous mandibles. Int J Oral Maxillofac Implants 1992;7:321–329.

9. Fugazzotto PA, Gulbransen HJ, Wheeler SL, Lindsay JA. The use of IMZ osseointegrated implants in partially and completely edentulous patients: Success and failure rates of 2023 implant cylinders up to 60+ months in function. Int J Oral Maxillofac Implants 1993;8:617–621.

10. Jemt T, Book K, Linden B, Urde G. Failures and complications in 92 consecutively inserted overdentures supported by Brånemark implants in severely resorbed edentulous maxillae; A study from prosthetic treatment to first annual checkup. Int J Oral Maxillofac Implants 1992;7:162–167.

11. Jemt T, Linden L, Lekholm U. Failures and complications in 127 consecutively placed fixed partial prostheses supported by Brånemark implants: From prosthetic treatment to first annual checkup. Int J Oral Maxillofac Implants 1992;7:40–44.

12. Sones AD. Complications with osseointegrated implants. J Prosthet Dent 1989;62:581–585.

13. Zarb GA, Schmitt A. The longitudinal clinical effectiveness of osseointegrated dental implants: The Toronto study. Part III: Problems and complications encountered. J Prosthet Dent 1990;64:185–194.

14. Johansson G, Palmquist S. Complications, supplementary treatment, and maintenance in edentulous arches with implant-supported fixed prostheses. Int J Prosthodont 1990;3:89–92.

15. Naert I, Quirynen M, van Steenberghe D, Darius P. A study of 589 consecutive implants supporting complete fixed prostheses. Part II: Prosthetic aspects. J Prosthet Dent 1992;68:949–956.

16. McGlumphy EA, Robinson DM, Mendel DA. Implant superstructures: A comparison of ultimate failure force. Int J Oral Maxillofac Implants 1992;7:35–39.

17. Tolman DE, Laney WR. Tissue-integrated prosthesis complications. Int J Oral Maxillofac Implants 1992;7:477–484.

18. Salonen MA, Oikarinen K, Virtanen K, Pernu H. Failures in the osseointegration of endosseous implants. Int J Oral Maxillofac Implants 1993;8:92–97.

19. Walton JN, MacEntee MI. Problems with prostheses on implants: A retrospective study. J Prosthet Dent 1994;71:283–288.

20. Kallus T, Bessing C. Loose gold screws frequently occur in full-arch fixed prostheses supported by osseointegrated implants after 5 years. Int J Oral Maxillofac Implants 1994;9:169–178.

21. Jemt T. Fixed implant-supported prostheses in the edentulous maxilla. A five-year follow-up report. Clin Oral Implants Res 1994;5:142–147.

22. Lekholm U, van Steenberghe D, Herrmann I, et al. Osseointegrated implants in the treatment of partially edentulous jaws. A prospective 5-year multicenter study. Int J Oral Maxillofac Implants 1994;9:627–635.

23. Carlson B, Carlsson GE. Prosthodontic complications in osseointegrated dental implant treatment. Int J Oral Maxillofac Implants 1994;9:90–94.

24. Hemmings KW, Schmitt A, Zarb GA. Complications and maintenance requirements for fixed prostheses and overdentures in the edentulous mandible: A 5-year report. Int J Oral Maxillofac Implants 1994;9:191–196.

25. Wie H. Registration of localization, occlusion and occluding materials for failing screw-joints in the Brånemark implant system. Clin Oral Implants Res 1995;6:47–53.

26. Rangert B, Jemt T, Jörneus L. Forces and moments on Brånemark implants. Int J Oral Maxillofac Implants 1989;4:241–247.

27. Jörneus L, Jemt T, Carlsson L. Loads and designs of screw joints for single crowns supported by osseointegrated implants. Int J Oral Maxillofac Implants 1992;7:353–359.

28. Rangert BR, Sullivan D, Jemt T. Load factor control for implants in the posterior partially edentulous segment. Int J Oral Maxillofac Implants 1997;12:360–370.

29. Bickford JH. An Introduction to the Design and Behavior of Bolted Joints. New York: Marcel Dekker, 1995.

30. Sakaguchi RL, Borgersen SE. Nonlinear finite element contact analysis of dental implant components. Int J Oral Maxillofac Implants 1993;8:655–661.

31. Haack JE, Sakaguchi RL, Sun T, Coffey JP. Elongation and preload stress in dental implant abutment screws. Int J Oral Maxillofac Implants 1993;10:529–536.

32. Weinberg LA. The biomechanics of force distribution in implant-supported prostheses. Int J Oral Maxillofac Implants 1993;8:19–31.

33. Brunski JB, Puleo DA, Nanci A. Biomaterials and biomechanics of oral and maxillofacial implants: Current status and future developments. Int J Oral Maxillofac Implants 2000;15:15–46.

34. Patterson EA, Johns RB. Theoretical analysis of the fatigue life of fixture screws in osseointegrated dental implants. Int J Oral Maxillofac Implants 1992;7(1):26–33.

35. McGlumphy EA, Mendel DA, Holloway JA. Implant screw mechanics. Dent Clin North Am 1998;42:71–89.

36. Lekholm U, Torsten J. Principles for single tooth replacement. In: Albrektsson T, Zarb GA (eds). The Brånemark Osseointegrated Implant. Chicago: Quintessence, 1989:117–126.

37. Laney WR, Tolman, DE. The Mayo Clinic experience with tissue-integrated prostheses. In: Albrektsson T, Zarb GA (eds). The Brånemark Osseointegrated Implant. Chicago: Quintessence, 1989:165–195.

38. Hobo S, Ichida E, Garcia LT. Osseointegration and Occlusal Rehabilitation. Chicago: Quintessence, 1989:65–73.

39. Ericsson I, Brånemark P-I, Glantz P-O. Partial edentulism. In: Worthington P, Brånemark P-I (eds). Advanced Osseointegration Surgery: Applications in the Maxillofacial Region. Chicago: Quintessence, 1992:194–209.

40. Ohrnell L-O, Palmquist J, Brånemark P-I. Single tooth replacement. In: Worthington P, Brånemark P-I (eds). Advanced Osseointegration Surgery: Applications in the Maxillofacial Region. Chicago: Quintessence, 1992:194–209.

41. Engquist B. Overdentures. In: Worthington P, Brånemark P-I (eds). Advanced Osseointegration Surgery: Applications in the Maxillofacial Region. Chicago: Quintessence, 1992:233–247.

42. Lang BR, Razzoog ME. Lingualized integration: Tooth molds and an occlusal scheme for edentulous implant patients. Implant Dent 1992;1:204–211.

43. Haraldson T, Zarb GA. A 10-year follow-up study of the masticatory system after treatment with osseointegrated implant bridges. Scand J Dent Res 1988;96(3):24–52.

44. Michael CG, Javid NS, Colaizzi FA, Gibbs CH. Biting strength and chewing forces in complete denture wearers. J Prosthet Dent 1990;63:549–553.

chapter 8

Implants in the Esthetic Zone

Robert B. O'Neal, DMD, MS, MEd

Treatment planning for the use of implants in the esthetic zone requires consideration of many factors and is a cooperative effort between the restorative dentist, the surgeon, and the dental technician. While the predictability of implants has greatly improved, facilitation of a favorable esthetic result remains a challenge for all involved. This chapter discusses many issues associated with the treatment planning of such cases and provides options for enhancing their success.

The use of dental implants to replace anterior teeth is one of the last areas to gain full acceptance by the dental profession. Reasons for this recent acceptance include improved presurgical planning guidelines, more options in the diameter of implants, greater variety of abutments, improved surgical guides to facilitate accurate placement of the implant, better techniques for preserving the soft tissue and preparing the edentulous site, and improved laboratory techniques. The cost of a single implant is comparable to that of a fixed partial denture, but the preparation of an edentulous site adds to costs in time and money for implant rehabilitation compared with conventional fixed partial denture prosthodontics. The dentist and the patient expect an anterior tooth replacement to be predictable and esthetic.[1] With current surgical and prosthodontic techniques, anterior restorations can be fabricated to meet these expectations.

The replacement of anterior teeth with implants provides a broad range of treatment planning options. When presented with the risks and benefits of all the available types of anterior tooth replacements, many patients choose the implant. The greatest benefit of using implants is the avoidance of unnecessary preparation of teeth adjacent to the implant site. Today, a well-informed patient may seek a second opinion if fixed or removable partial dentures are the only options a dentist provides. Furthermore, failure to inform a patient that an implant is an option is considered in many areas of the world to be practicing be-

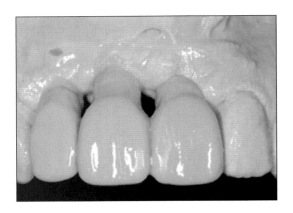

Fig 8-1 Significant ridge resorption and loss of papillae may be corrected more predictably with conventional prosthodontic restorations. (Reprinted from O'Neal and Butler[5] with permission.)

neath the standard of care regarding informed consent.

The replacement and restoration of anterior teeth with implants should be incorporated into a practice only after the surgeon and the restoring dentist have gained considerable experience with implants in nonesthetic areas.[2,3] The use of study casts, a diagnostic waxup, and proper radiographs early in the treatment planning stage can greatly aid in choosing the proper treatment.[4] An ideally shaped partially edentulous ridge, better preserved papillae, and a waxup of the tooth that matches the natural shape of the adjacent teeth will all result in more predictable implant treatment. When more than one anterior tooth is missing, there is a characteristic shrinkage of the ridge, with flattening or complete loss of the papillae between the missing teeth. This type of ridge defect may be restored more predictably with conventional prosthodontics (Fig 8-1).

Correction of Compromised Edentulous Sites

Although some anterior teeth are congenitally missing, most missing anterior teeth are extracted secondary to trauma, endodontic complication, fracture, periodontal disease, or caries. Rarely are these anterior edentulous sites without some compromise in the width and height of the edentulous ridge, gingival papillae height, or thickness of the overlying gingivae.[6,7] Implants in the esthetic zone (Figs 8-2a to 8-2f) may require ridge augmentation. Whether an implant or fixed partial denture is used, most ridge defects need correction to achieve acceptable esthetics.[6,8] Patients with thick gingiva, thick alveolar bone, and square-shaped teeth tend to have less resorption of the remaining ridge than do patients with thin gingiva, thin bone, and a tapered tooth shape.[9] A high smile line revealing gingival display

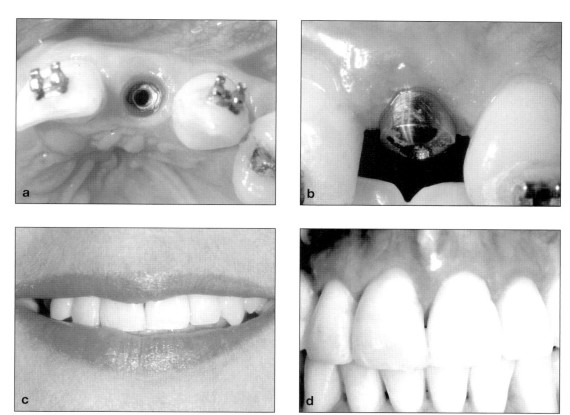

Figs 8-2a to 8-2d Ideal placement of implants is essential in the esthetic zone. (Reprinted from O'Neal and Butler[5] with permission.)

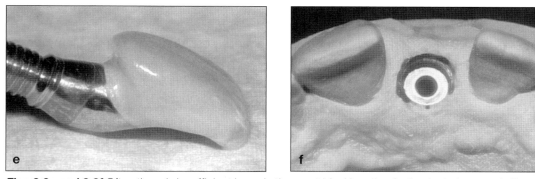

Figs 8-2e and 8-2f Often there is insufficient bone in the most ideal location for implant placement. One approach to solving this problem is the fabrication of a ridge-lap crown. However, this type of restoration complicates hygiene procedures. (Reprinted from O'Neal and Butler[5] with permission.)

with a thin gingival architecture presents more of a challenge in achieving esthetic results.

Augmentation at the time of extraction

Ridge preservation and augmentation at the time of extraction can greatly increase the esthetic appeal of an implant-restored tooth. Procedures that can be used at this time are atraumatic extraction followed by debridement of the socket and grafting with alloplastic, allogeneic, and/or autogenous materials; guided bone regeneration with membranes; orthodontic extrusion of the root prior to extraction; and the use of an ovate pontic for development of gingival contours.

Implants have significantly changed both staging and techniques for the extraction of teeth that are potential sites for implant placement. The ability to make some critical treatment planning decisions prior to extraction of the tooth can produce a more esthetic outcome and reduce cost for the patient. Factors to consider are the contours of the gingival margin and the papillae from the corners of the smile, which in some cases may extend to the first molar. Every effort should be taken to preserve the gingival tissues and avoid any compromise in the bone surrounding the socket or the adjacent teeth. When extracting a tooth, the gingival tissues should be detached from the tooth with a sharp scalpel incision. If forceps are used for the extraction, the clinician should avoid any compromise of the gingival tissues and crestal and buccal plates of the remaining socket bone. Many clinicians are using a thin-bladed instrument (periotome) to extract single-rooted teeth, especially when there is inadequate tooth structure for the forceps to secure the root without damage to the tissue or bone (Fig 8-3). The apical area of the extraction socket must be meticulously debrided of all granulation tissue, as this residual tissue may prevent or delay healing of the socket with mature bone.

Anterior teeth that are facially prominent or that have a thin facial alveolar plate of bone can heal with a significant ridge deformity (Fig 8-4). There is a trend to graft the extraction socket in the hopes of reducing the degree of alveolar ridge resorption. This technique needs further long-term evaluation before it can be routinely recommended. Presently there are many biocompatible resorbable materials available for grafting the alveolar socket; none has shown significant superiority over the other. Autogenous grafting material is still the gold standard.

Prevention of ridge resorption can be accomplished in several ways that are more predictable. If there is loss of the facial plate of the socket, the use of guided bone regeneration procedures, ie, placement of barrier membranes along with bone grafting materials, is beneficial. A facial full-thickness flap is reflected and the socket is filled with a resorbable grafting material. A barrier membrane is placed over the graft material. It provides support to reestablish ridge contour, holds the graft in place, and prevents soft tissue of the gingival flap from collapsing into the socket. The major disadvantage to the procedure is the need to coronally position the flap to obtain primary coverage of the barrier membrane. This can create an unesthetic change in the mucogingival line, which can, however, be corrected at the time of implant placement.

Another method of preventing ridge resorption is through orthodontic extrusion

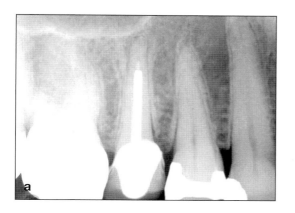

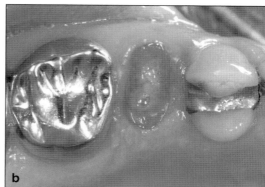

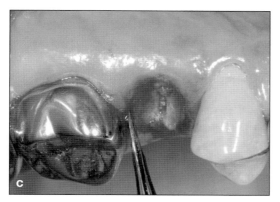

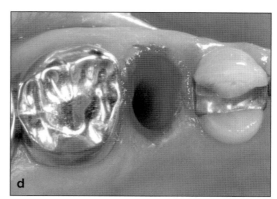

Fig 8-3 Implants have significantly changed both staging and techniques for extracting teeth that are potential sites for implant placement and fixed denture pontics. The ability to make some critical treatment planning decisions prior to extraction of the tooth can produce a more esthetic outcome and reduce both cost and time for the patient. Every effort is now taken to preserve the gingival tissues and avoid any compromise in the bone surrounding the socket. (Reprinted from O'Neal and Butler[5] with permission.) *(a)* Endodontically treated roots are difficult to extract without risk of fracturing the crown and dislodging the post. *(b)* Remaining roots should be extracted without sacrificing gingiva and alveolar bone. *(c)* The periotome is a thin-bladed instrument placed within the periodontal ligament space, with pressure alternating mesially and distally, without twisting, until the remaining root becomes mobile. *(d)* The root can be removed with minimal trauma to the surrounding gingival tissues and without sacrificing the buccal shelf of alveolar bone. *(e)* Periotomes are available in both straight and angled configurations.

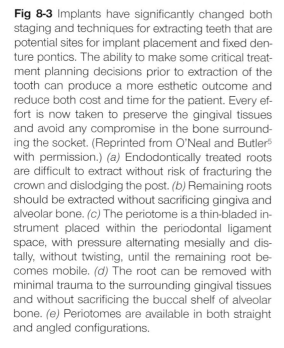

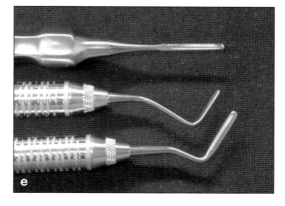

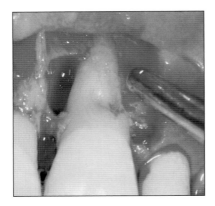

Fig 8-4 Following extraction, sites that once held periodontally involved teeth or teeth that were fractured below the crestal bone normally heal with a significantly compromised ridge. Complete loss of the labial plate and mesial interproximal alveolar bone make this site ideal for grafting at the time of extraction. (Reprinted from O'Neal and Butler[5] with permission.)

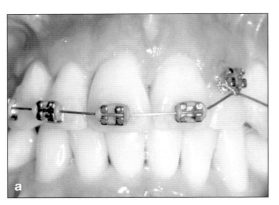

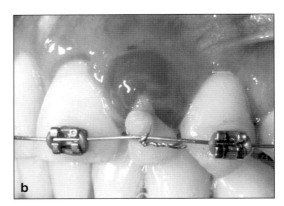

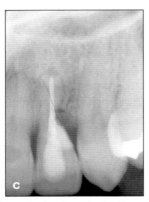

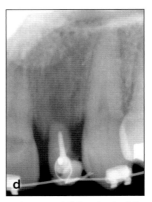

Fig 8-5 Prior to extraction of a tooth with significant bone loss and thin gingival tissues, orthodontic extrusion should be considered. (Reprinted from O'Neal and Butler[5] with permission.) *(a)* The bracket should be placed as close as possible to the gingiva to allow for maximum extrusion. *(b)* The tooth should be shortened continually as it is extruded. The bracket can be apically repositioned or replaced with a custom button until the desired extrusion has been accomplished. The dark tissue is the original pocket epithelium that evaginated during the extrusion process. *(c)* Radiograph prior to orthodontic extrusion. The root had external resorption and upon probing was found to be within 3 mm of the apex facially. *(d)* The remaining root tip after orthodontic extrusion. Note that the interproximal bone of the root tip is more coronal than that of the adjacent teeth.

Box 8-1 Methods for edentulous ridge development

1. Connective tissue grafts
2. Ridge expansion
3. Bone grafting of ridge deformities
   - With autogenous donor tissue
     - Block or particle grafts
     - Chin, ramus, edentulous ridge, or iliac crest
   - With other grafting materials
     - Allografts
     - Xenografts
     - Synthetic substances
   - With other promising materials
     - Platelet-rich plasma (PRP) concentrate
     - Bone morphogenetic proteins (BMPs)
4. Guided bone regeneration
   - With resorbable and/or nonresorbable membranes
   - With or without grafting materials

---

for site development. Orthodontic extrusion of the remaining root provides two significant advantages to site development (Fig 8-5). *(1)* Both bone and soft tissue are coronally positioned. The additional bone and soft tissue enhance the site for a more esthetic final restoration. *(2)* With orthodontic extrusion, the diameter of the remaining socket becomes much smaller, and many times an implant can be placed in this socket at the time of extraction.

Placement of a temporary crown/pontic that is contoured to preserve or establish the gingival contours is a critical step in site development. Prior to the extraction, fabrication of a provisional prosthesis with an ovate crown/pontic rather than a ridge-lap design is recommended, because the ovate design can help preserve the form of dental papillae and facial gingival contour, allowing for more ideal contour of the implant-

supported restoration. Care must be taken not to overcontour the ovate crown/pontic and cause facial recession or displace the interproximal papillae.

Edentulous ridge development must be performed if either *(1)* bone is deficient for implant placement or *(2)* gingival contours are inadequate for the final restoration. There are four general methods for accomplishing this (Box 8-1).

Augmentation of healed extraction sites

Unfortunately, in many instances, extractions of anterior teeth are performed well before an implant has been planned for its replacement. Many of these edentulous sites have healed with a hard or soft tissue ridge deformity. This residual ridge can compromise or contraindicate the placement of

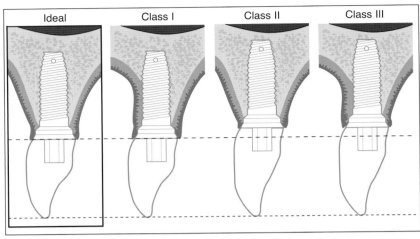

Fig 8-6 Classification of ridge deformities. *(left to right)* Ideal ridge with minimal resorption of the labial width or height of the ridges; Class I: loss of width would leave threads of the implant exposed or the implant would need to be placed too far palatally; Class II: loss of height of the ridge would create a longer than normal crown; Class III: loss of width and height would make for a long crown, and the implant would be placed far to the palatal to avoid thread exposure. (Illustration by David W. Ehlert. Courtesy of University of Washington, Seattle, WA.)

an implant and/or the esthetic restoration of an implant. A tooth with a vertical fracture buccolingually through the root can destroy the entire buccal plate of bone and, in some cases, the palatal plate as well. A number of techniques have been developed to regenerate lost hard and soft tissue.[10]

The use of a surgical/radiographic guide based on appropriate radiographs and the initial waxup of the missing tooth is critical. These aids help determine the ideal location of the implant, the diameter of implant needed, and the depth of placement as it relates to the anticipated emergence profile and contours of the abutment and final restoration. With this information, the surgeon and the restorative dentist can determine whether or not there is adequate hard and soft tissue to place an implant in the ideal location, what type of ridge deformity exists, and what steps need to be taken to create a suitable bed into which an implant can be placed to achieve an acceptable outcome.

Treatment of specific ridge deformities

There are three classifications of ridge deformities (Fig 8-6). A Class I ridge deformity is the loss of buccolingual width without loss of ridge height, Class II is the loss of coronal ridge height, and Class III is a combination of Class I and II.[11] Class II and III ridge defects are difficult to augment, and the consistency of achieving an ideal esthetic result is unpredictable. Fortunately, the majority of ridge defects are Class I.[2] In a Class I ridge, there

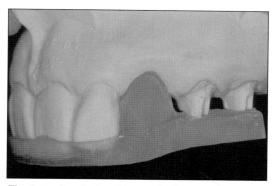

Fig 8-7a Surgical guide made from a diagnostic waxup showing the desired tooth shape and location of the gingival margin.

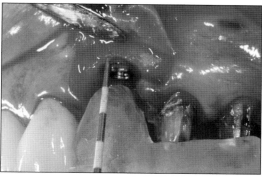

Fig 8-7b The use of a surgical guide ensures proper placement as well as proper depth for an ideal emergence profile. Normally, the implant should be placed 3 to 4 mm below the cemento-enamel junction of the adjacent teeth.

should be at least 6 mm of ridge width and an acceptable height of the ridge to place a standard 3.75- or 4.0-mm-diameter implant. The height of the ridge should be such that the implant will be approximately 3 to 4 mm apical to the cementoenamel junction of the adjacent teeth. This allows for proper emergence profile and contour of the crown from the top of the implant (Figs 8-7a and 8-7b). Larger-diameter implants can be used where the ridge width and mesiodistal distance are adequate and where there is space for interproximal bone between the adjacent teeth and the implant. The gingival contours should be acceptable and fill the embrasures between the implant crown and the adjacent teeth. Recent studies have demonstrated that the tip of the papillae normally will be about 5 mm from the crest of the interproximal bone.[3] Preservation of the crestal bone height adjacent to the other teeth is critical at the time of extraction as well at the time of implant placement.

When the edentulous ridge and/or the soft tissue contours prove to be insufficient

in the diagnostic waxup, soft tissue and/or bone-regenerating techniques need to be considered. The horizontal Class I ridge defects are predictable to treat. These techniques add additional time and cost to the procedure but still avoid preparation of the adjacent teeth.

In Class I ridge deformities, the bone volume may be adequate to place the implant at the ideal location, and only augmentation of the ridge with a connective tissue graft over the facial bone or over the implant is needed to enhance the tissue contours. In some cases, particulate grafting material can be used to enhance the final alveolar bone contours prior to placement of the connective tissue graft. The ridge can also be split mesiodistally using a fine-blade chisel. The facial bone can be slightly displaced at the time of implant placement through the use of osteotomes.

Augmentation to correct for Class II and III ridge deformities using barrier membranes and/or grafting materials is becoming predictable. Augmentation is technique

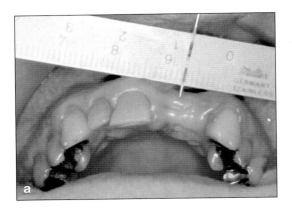
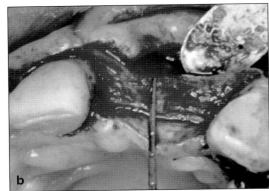
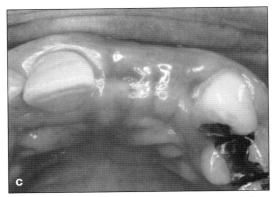
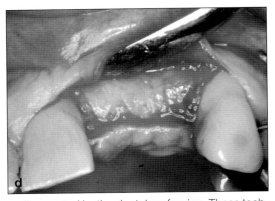

Fig 8-8 Techniques for regenerating bone have become well accepted by the dental profession. These techniques do add additional time and cost to implant treatment but still avoid preparation of the adjacent teeth, which would be required if conventional fixed partial denture treatment were to be performed. (Reprinted from O'Neal and Butler[5] with permission.) *(a)* The alveolar ridge has a large facial concavity. *(b)* The alveolar bone is too thin faciopalatally for implant placement, unless the implant is placed palatally. *(c)* The alveolar ridge after grafting, without the facial concavity. *(d)* The width of the alveolar ridge has been increased, allowing an implant to be placed in an ideal location.

sensitive, but the results allow ideal implant placement. The use of these techniques can add 6 months or more to the total time before the final restoration can be placed. The use of barrier membranes over block grafts or bone grafting materials contoured to the ideal ridge contours is the most predictable approach to implant site development (Fig 8-8). Many clinicians are adding a concentrate of platelets (PRP) derived from the patient's own blood to the grafting material to enhance platelet-derived growth factors at the healing site. Research on the PRP technique is ongoing, as is that on the addition of BMPs derived from animal sources or produced synthetically. The theory behind both of these approaches is to provide growth factors in a concentration that is high enough to stimulate and accelerate growth.

Restorative Procedures

Provisional restoration

Provisional restorations that can be adjusted and contoured are critical to establish proper gingival contours prior to fabrication of the final restoration. The standard protocol is to make an impression of the implant after the area of implant placement is well healed. Many clinicians, however, make an index of the implant at the time of placement, rather than waiting 6 months. This index of the implant is keyed to the adjacent teeth. Most manufacturers provide a variety of prefabricated abutments plus an index impression coping that allows for fabrication of a custom abutment. With the indexed cast, the restoring dentist can then choose an abutment and fabricate a provisional restoration; these can then be ready at the time the implant is exposed at stage 2 surgery. The most ideal approach is to place a small healing abutment at stage 2 to allow maximum soft tissue adaptation around the abutment and interproximally. Once the tissues have healed, a screw-retained provisional crown is much easier to use for customizing the contours of the provisional restoration. A provisional crown can be modified by adding or recontouring it over several appointments in the development of ideal tissue contours prior to the making the final restoration. This approach is more expensive and time consuming, but the result achieved is well worth the extra effort.

Final restoration

The final crown can either be screw-retained or cemented over the abutment. Most anterior crowns are cemented with temporary cement. The use of temporary cement allows the crown to be removed in the future if needed. However, the disadvantage of this technique is that cement may be trapped subgingivally, especially if the margin is 3 to 4 mm subgingival. If the cement is not completely removed, gingival inflammation may occur. Further, the crown may on occasion become loose at inopportune times.

Summary

There are numerous articles in the literature that address diagnosis and treatment planning of implant restorations in the esthetic zone. Articles on techniques for improving placement of the implant, ridge enhancement, indexing the implant, and improving tissue contours are published almost monthly. Unfortunately, many of these articles are based on case reports with limited long-term follow-up. Well-controlled prospective studies are strongly needed to help the profession better treat patients who seek our care.

References

1. Chang M, Odman PA, Wennstrom JL, Andersson B. Esthetic outcome of implant-supported single-tooth replacements assessed by the patient and by prosthodontists. Int J Prosthodont 1999;12:335–341.
2. American Academy of Periodontology. Position paper: Dental implants in periodontal therapy. J Periodontol 2000;71:1934–1942.
3. Weisgold AS, Arnoux JP, Lu J. Single-tooth anterior implant: A world of caution. Part I. J Esthet Dent 1997;9:225–233.

4. Hess D, Buser D, Dietschi D, Grossen G, Schonenberger A, Belzer UC. Esthetic single-tooth replacement with implants: A team approach. Quintessence Int 1998;29:77–86.

5. O'Neal RB, Butler B. Restoration or implant placement: A growing treatment quandary. Periodontol 2000 2002;30:111–122.

6. Abrams H, Kopczyck RA, Kaplan AL. Incidence of anterior ridge deformities in partially edentulous patients. J Prosthet Dent 1987;57:191–194.

7. Choquet V, Hermans M, Adriaenssens P, Daelemans P, Tarnow DP, Malevez C. Clinical and radiographic evaluation of the papilla level adjacent to single-tooth dental implants. A retrospective study in the maxillary anterior region. J Periodontol 2001;72:1364–1371.

8. Widmark G, Andersson B, Ivanoff CJ. Mandibular bone graft in the anterior maxilla for single-tooth implants. Presentation of surgical method. Int J Oral Maxillofac Surg 1997;26:106–109.

9. Nemcovsky CE, Moses O, Artzi Z. Interproximal papillae reconstruction in maxillary implants. J Periodontol 2000;71:308–314.

10. Bahat O, Fontanessi RV. Implant placement in three-dimensional grafts in the anterior jaw. Int J Periodontics Restorative Dent 2001;21:357–365.

11. Seibert J. Reconstruction of deformed partial edentulous ridges using full-thickness onlay grafts. Part II. Compend Contin Educ Dent 1983; 4:549–562.

chapter 9

Maintenance

Michael E. Razzoog, DDS, MS, MPH
Lars G. Hollender, DDS

There are four elements in the maintenance program for the patient with dental implants. First is the establishment of a home-care regimen in personal oral hygiene that helps the patient achieve an acceptable level of plaque control. The second element is reinforcement of this regimen by periodic recall appointments, which evaluate the patient's progress and monitor the status of the implants and the health of the supporting tissues. Strict adherence to a recall schedule, along with verification that the implant prosthesis continues to satisfy the requirements of function, comfort, and esthetics initially established, is the third element in the maintenance program. The fourth element is a lifetime commitment by the patient to the tenets of the maintenance program; this is the overriding factor in long-term prosthetic implant success.

Oral Hygiene Home-Care Regimen

Meticulous home care must be demonstrated by the patient during the presurgical phase of treatment. To ensure good oral hygiene, the daily home-care program of the patient must be customized to the individual's ability to keep plaque off the remaining natural teeth. Emphasis must be directed toward the proper use of a toothbrush and the use of dental floss to clean debris from around the remaining natural teeth.[1,2]

After placement of the implants in stage 1 surgery, hygiene recall visits at appropriate intervals will be needed to monitor plaque control and to prevent the occurrence of an inflammatory response in the tissues around the natural teeth and in the area of the implants.

Uncovering of the implants and placement of the abutment components during stage 2 surgery necessitates additional home-care considerations. The sutures used in the tissues adjacent to the abutment make it somewhat difficult to maintain oral hygiene. There is the tendency for patients to be afraid of damaging their implants and thus to be less aggressive in oral hygiene measures than is necessary. Additional instruction in oral hygiene techniques with soft toothbrushes and end-tufted brushes can help patients keep the implant abutments clean. A number of interdental devices, including specialized flossing materials and oral irrigation devices, have been designed for cleaning the interproximal areas of teeth. If available, these devices should be used on both the natural teeth and the abutment surfaces, where they have proven equally beneficial in removing plaque.

Chlorhexidine, an antimicrobial agent, may be prescribed as an oral rinse to reduce the adherence of plaque to the surface of the implant abutment. However, rinsing must stop when the implant prosthesis is attached to the abutment, because the solution will stain the artificial teeth and base materials of the prosthesis.[3] Instead, the chlorhexidine should be applied around the abutments with a brush or cotton-tipped swab to minimize staining and maximize the concentration of the agent at the soft tissue–abutment interface.

Regardless of the technique or device that is used by the patient in customizing the home-care program, plaque removal from teeth and the implant abutments is the ultimate goal.

Reinforcement of Home Care at the Recall Appointment

Reinforcement of the home-care program by periodic recall appointments to evaluate the status of the implants and the health of the supporting tissues is essential to the success of implant treatment. A recall appointment schedule must be set up following placement of the prosthesis and completion of the initial phases of prosthodontic treatment.

During the first year following placement of the implant prosthesis, the patient should be seen every 3 to 4 months. After the first year, the patient should be placed on a recall schedule that meets the individual's needs; however, 6 months between recall appointments should be the longest interval considered for the patient with dental implants.

At each recall appointment, the dentist must assess the tissue surrounding the implant abutment. The dentist should consider any deviation in color and consistency from the state of health routinely observed about a sound implant abutment. In addition, spontaneous bleeding or bleeding induced by a toothbrush must be recorded in the patient's chart. Tissue surrounding the implant should appear light pink or coral in color and be firm and resilient. Marginal gingiva around the abutment will usually taper to a knife-edge junction next to the abutment or the implant restoration. Probing of pocket depth, a commonly accepted measurement in the monitoring of the health of the periodontium around natural teeth, is sometimes used to evaluate the tissue-abutment interface. If a probe is to be used, it must be made of plastic to protect the abutment from being scratched.

Status of Implants at the Recall Appointment

The overall success of dental rehabilitation with an implant-supported prosthesis depends on continuous stability of the prosthesis, which in turn depends on the long-term anchorage of the individual implants. The maintenance of osseointegration along the entire implant surface and of marginal bone height along the vertical extent of the implant are the two factors necessary for proper implant anchorage. Both of these factors depend on local stress concentrations; the marginal bone height is also influenced by reactions in the marginal soft tissues around the implant.

The even distribution of stress among all the implants will contribute favorably to the maintenance of marginal bone close to the implants. The accuracy of fit of the prosthesis to the implants should be checked at recall examinations. Undue or uneven forces on the bone may lead to microfractures that could elicit the development of nonmineralized connective tissue. Optimization of stress distribution is of continuing importance in implant prosthodontics.

Some bone loss will be noted at recall examinations. Reports in the literature suggest that 1 to 1.5 mm of marginal bone is lost during the first year after connection of the prosthesis to the implants, mainly in response to the surgical trauma.[4] Subsequent annual marginal bone loss after the first year is around 0.05 to 0.1 mm. Therefore, a bone loss of less than 0.1 mm per year appears to be routine. This represents a loss of about 2 mm of vertical bone support during the first 10 years following implant placement.

The 1978 Harvard Conference on dental implants concluded that implant survival rates in maxillae and mandibles were approximately 85% and 95%, respectively.[5] It would appear that it is more difficult to achieve and maintain osseointegration in maxillae than in mandibles. It was also reported that the majority of implant losses occur during the first year. Recall examinations are thus extremely important for ensuring the long-term success of osseointegrated implants.

Oral prophylaxis for the implant patient

Certain modifications in oral prophylactic procedures involving osseointegrated dental implants are necessary during recall appointments. Conventional metal instruments and ultrasonic cleaning devices may scratch the titanium components and/or loosen retention screws.[6] Plastic cleaning instruments that conform to the implant surface when properly positioned by the operator and that prevent abrasion of the implant abutment should be used instead.

For those situations in which calculus cannot be removed with plastic instruments, the careful use of an air-powder–abrasive system may be indicated. Several of these machines are available, and although expensive, they are valuable in the removal of calculus from inaccessible places.

Radiographic monitoring

The principles of postimplantation imaging are not different from those applied for the radiographic examinations of the ordinary dental patient (see chapter 3). However, there seems to be a documented need for checking the fit between abutment and implant after abutment connection. This is best done using intraoral radiographic film

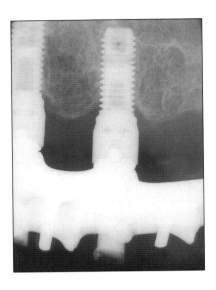

Fig 9-1 Follow-up intraoral radiograph with an optimal projection disclosing the threading of the implant on both sides.

with a beam direction that is favorable for detecting a misfit between implant and abutment. Individual images may be required for optimal assessment of individual implants. If implants are threaded, an optimal image would show the threads clearly and equally depicted on both sides of the implant (Fig 9-1). Deviations from the ideal beam direction will result in overlap of the threads, creating a diffuse image of them, and one side will show more "blurring" or overlap than the other, depending on the direction of the beam. For standard threaded implants, the left side of the implant will show more overlap when the radiation is directed from below versus the ideal beam direction. This means that implants in the maxilla will show more overlap on the right side than the left if the beam was directed from above the ideal beam direction.

Radiographic examination may also be warranted when the implant prosthesis is placed to check the fit between the compo-

nents, including that between implant and abutment.

Repeated radiographic examinations of implants are not warranted, but a 1-year follow-up examination to establish the level of the alveolar bone around the implants appears to be desirable. Thereafter, clinical signs and symptoms should govern the timing of radiographic examinations; there seems to be no need for annual radiographic examinations.

In a few cases there may be a need for a three-dimensional evaluation of an implant, for instance, to demonstrate the relationship between the implant and critical anatomic structures, such as the mandibular canal, or if the implant has perforated the cortical plate of the bone on the buccal or lingual side (Figs 9-2a to 9-2c). Conventional tomography may then be the modality of choice, since the metallic implant may prevent successful imaging with computerized tomography (CT) (see Figs 9-2b and 9-2c).

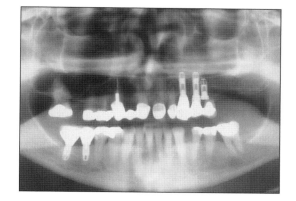

Fig 9-2a Panoramic radiograph of a patient with two implants in the mandible and symptoms of paresthesia and numbness.

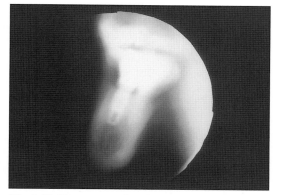

Fig 9-2b Tomogram showing the anterior implant above the mandibular canal.

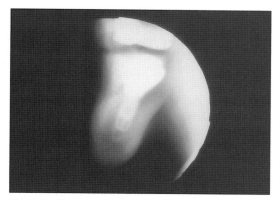

Fig 9-2c Tomogram showing the posterior implant placed partially into the mandibular canal.

A successful implant is characterized by an unchanged level of the crestal bone after the initial bone loss (ie, the 1.0 to 1.5 mm of loss that may take place in the first year after an implant is placed). Many times bone is formed around the implant. Radiographically, this can be seen as a fine radiopaque line parallel to the implant (Fig 9-3). This line denotes the outer border of this new bone formation but is not seen in all cases.

Failure of implants at an early stage is usually seen radiographically via a radiolu-cent zone along the implant borders. However, such radiolucent zones can be created by so-called Mach band effects. Implants that fail in later stages usually show increasing bone loss at the alveolar margin. Many times this bone loss produces V-shaped defects around the implant. Such bony defects can also be seen in conjunction with implant fractures (Figs 9-4a and 9-4b). Many of these fractures occur at the level of the abutment screw. In rare instances periapical osteolytic changes occur.

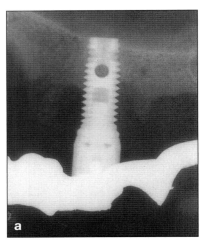 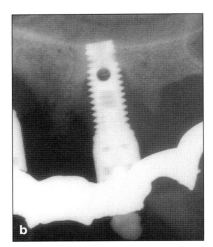

Fig 9-3 Follow-up intraoral radiographs taken 8 months apart demonstrating progressive bone loss around a maxillary implant.

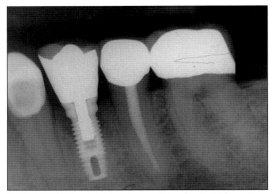 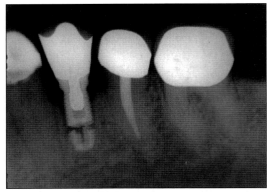

Fig 9-4a Follow-up intraoral radiograph showing bone loss along the implant to the level of the abutment screw.

Fig 9-4b Radiograph taken 6 months later showing a horizontal fracture below the abutment screw.

In patients in whom bone has been transplanted on the buccal or lingual surfaces of the alveolar process, ordinary periapical radiographs serve little purpose to disclose failure or success. In such cases, tomography or CT, or sometimes occlusal radiographs, should be employed. The outcome of sinus lift procedures can be studied by intraoral and panoramic radiographs, but CT is probably needed to demonstrate unequivocally whether the transplanted bone has successfully integrated with the border of the maxillary sinus. In cases where a radiolucent space seems to separate the transplanted bone from the border of the maxillary sinus, one has to consider the possibility that the transplanted bone is separated from the host bone by soft tissue.

Status of Implant Prosthesis at the Recall Appointment

The conditions seen most frequently during periodic recall appointments that require attention are gingivitis, soft tissue hyperplasia, small fistulae, exposed implant threads, fracture of the abutment screw, fracture of the anchorage mechanism between the prosthesis and the abutment, loss of optimal occlusal contacts, and fracture of the prosthodontic framework.

Loosening of implant components is the most frequently encountered condition; this underlines the importance of accurate fit between implant components, especially at the prosthodontic interface. Tightening the screws will correct the condition temporarily; however, should the condition recur, careful attention should be given to the accuracy of fit. Fracture of the abutment screw, fracture of the gold screw, and late loss of the implant are rare occurrences, but they also may be related to lack of a precise fit between the implant components and the prosthesis.

If the components are not loose and the patient is demonstrating reasonable oral hygiene, then no obvious advantage can be gained from the removal of the prosthesis. However, the oral condition may be such that removal of the prosthesis is necessary to clean around the abutments. Most implant components from different manufacturers are not interchangeable, so the dentist must have on hand the appropriate components and instrumentation for the implant system used for the patient.

Cleaning of the removed prosthesis is easily accomplished using an ultrasonic cleaning device. If the prosthesis requires instrumentation to remove tenacious calculus or to polish the metal surfaces, the metal components at the prosthodontic interface must be covered with laboratory protective caps or brass analogs. All dental personnel must exercise the greatest of care when cleaning these areas with instruments and polishing agents to avoid damage to the prosthodontic interface.

With the prosthesis removed, the abutment should be examined for looseness and tightened, if necessary, using the appropriate instrumentation. Experience has shown that loose abutment screws are responsible for most of the adverse tissue responses surrounding the abutment at recall appointments, including hyperplasia, hypertrophy, and progressive marginal bone loss.

There should be no space at the prosthodontic interface. If a space is seen, the exact cause for the change must be determined and corrected. Simply replacing the prosthesis and tightening the screws will ultimately lead to further complications and possible implant loss.

Excess forces resulting from malocclusion may also contribute to the early loss of an implant. At every recall appointment, the restorative dentist must evaluate the occlusal contacts in centric and eccentric positions, looking for changes that have occurred as a result of wear or other factors. If corrections are necessary, they must be performed.

Lifetime Commitment to Maintenance

To prevent complications with dental implant treatment, the dentist must establish a healthy oral environment and the patient must aid in long-term implant maintenance. The patient must become a co-therapist and take a level of responsibility for his or her oral condition. This chapter has recommended a series of recall activities and strict protocols that have proven to be successful in promoting a continuous level of health. While these mechanisms are known to be helpful, the implant patient must be educated and encouraged to understand his or her role in the maintenance of implant health.

References

1. Beumer J III, Lewis SG. The Brånemark Implant System: Clinical and Laboratory Procedures. St Louis: Ishiyaku EuroAmerica, 1989:34–35, 100–103.
2. Hobo S, Ichida E, Garcia LT. Osseointegration and Occlusal Rehabilitation. Chicago: Quintessence, 1989:239–254.
3. Khokhar Z, Razzoog ME, Yaman P. Color stability of restorative resins. Quintessence Int 1991;22: 733–737.
4. Adell R, Lekholm U, Rockler B, Brånemark P-I. A 15-year study of osseointegrated implants in the treatment of the edentulous jaw. Int J Oral Surg 1987;10:387–416.
5. Schnitman PA, Shulman LB. Recommendations on the consensus development conference on dental implants. J Am Dent Assoc 1979;98: 373–377.
6. Thomson-Neal DM, Evans GH, Meffert RM, Davenport WD. An SEM evaluation of various prophylactic modalities on different implants. Int J Periodontics Restorative Dent 1989;9:301–311.

chapter 10

Complications and Failure

Philip Worthington, MD, BSc
Jeffrey E. Rubenstein, DMD, MS

Definitions of success, survival, and failure with dental implants have evolved over the years. It is now generally accepted that to be regarded as successful, an endosseous implant must do more than remain present in the jaw (Box 10-1).[1] It must also demonstrate clinical immobility under load-bearing conditions, and it should be free of associated symptoms such as discomfort, pain, and tenderness. There should be no impairment in the function of adjacent structures, such as the inferior alveolar nerve and its mental branch, natural tooth abutments, inferior alveolar nerve, or the sinus or nasal cavities. There should be no progressive, continuing radiolucency surrounding the implant, and loss of crestal bone height should be minimal. When failures occur they are usually, but not always, attributable to deviation from the procedures outlined in this text: patient selection may have been imprudent, planning may have been incomplete, consultation between clinicians may have been inadequate, or technique during the surgical,

> **Box 10-1** Criteria for success of endosseous implants
>
> - Clinical immobility
> - Ability to bear load
> - No associated symptoms
> - No damage to adjacent structures
> - No progressive peri-implant radiolucency
> - Minimal loss of crestal bone height

prosthetic, and laboratory phases of treatment may have been faulty.

Osseointegration may fail to develop, or having developed, may later be lost. The causes of failed osseointegration are not always known. In some instances, failure may be biologic, eg, the bone may be too avascular or perhaps inadequate in quantity, quality, and density. The failure may be iatrogenic, eg, the bone may have been overheated during implant site preparation. Osseointegration may be subsequently lost because of overloading, perhaps the result of inadequate prosthetic design, inaccuracy of fit, or a patient's parafunctional habits leading to overload and fatigue failure.

Indications of Failure

An implant that is persistently tender or that a patient says "just doesn't feel right" should be checked for failed osseointegration. If it is in the posterior mandible, then encroachment of the inferior alveolar nerve or possibly perforation, eg, of the lingual cortical plate, may have occurred. Mobility of an endosseous implant is a clear sign of failure, and the implant should be removed. The clinician needs to differentiate between an abutment screw that has loosened or fractured versus an implant that has either fractured or lost integration. The development of a peri-implant radiolucent line on a radiograph is not usually an early sign of failure, but when present it indicates that the bone has receded from the implant surface and that the intervening space has been occupied by granulation tissue or a fibrous tissue sheath. This indicates incomplete osseointegration and probable implant failure.

When an individual implant fails, the clinician should remove it and possibly allow the site to heal completely before considering placement of a new implant. Under special circumstances, the implant site may be cleaned of granulation and fibrous tissue, and an implant of greater diameter can be immediately placed.

Complications

Complications may result from biologic, iatrogenic, or mechanical factors. Biologic fac-

tors tending to produce complications include bone of poor quality or inadequate volume, smoking, and previous irradiation or immunosuppression. Iatrogenic factors include inappropriate case selection, faulty planning, deviation from recommended surgical protocol, and prosthodontic overloading due to poor design. Mechanical factors include overly forceful manipulation and patient parafunctional habits, such as bruxism.

Complications associated with implant placement

Faulty placement may take several forms. Implants may be placed too close together or be misaligned, resulting in challenges for abutment selection, spacing, and access for hygiene, as well as biomechanical compromise. Faulty angulation of implants may be avoided by care in planning and the use of surgical stents, which communicate to the surgeon or clinician who is placing the implants their anticipated desired position and inclination. Implants may be placed too close together, so that it is difficult to attach the abutments or keep the intervening mucosa healthy. They may be placed too far to the labial or buccal aspect of the jaw, which may result in exposure of the implant threads (Fig 10-1). This may be remedied by the use of bone grafts or guided tissue regeneration to build up bone volume. Similarly, implants placed too far lingually may suffer because of the thin, vulnerable, and mobile mucosa of the floor of the mouth. Faulty angulation of implants may be avoided by care in planning and the use of surgical templates and guides; and the condition may sometimes be remedied by the use of angulated abutments.

Excessive countersinking at the mouth of the implant site is to be avoided, especially

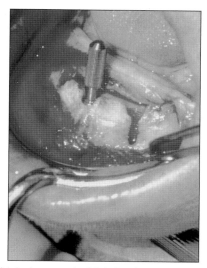

Fig 10-1 Labial placement of this implant resulted in exposure of the threads on the labial aspect. Had a template been used, this error might have been avoided.

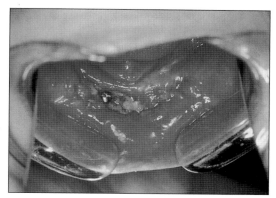

Fig 10-2 Dehiscence of the incision used for implant placement. In this instance, this was attributed to previous irradiation of the area during treatment of an oral carcinoma.

in the posterior mandible, where internal support for the implant may be lacking due to the loosely textured trabecular bone.

A damaged, eccentric, or badly handled drill may result in an ovoid, rather than circular, implant site cross section. The implant-bone contact is thus diminished, lessening the likelihood of successful osseointegration.

When bone is overheated during the preparation of the implant site, bone cells in the immediate vicinity of the interface may not survive. The bone may die back from the implant surface and be replaced by less differentiated scar tissue, making failure more likely. The use of sharp drills with intermittent and gentle pressure, drills of incremental sizes, copious coolant irrigation, and strictly controlled rotational drill speeds will minimize the risk of overheating.

Dehiscence of the soft tissue at the line of incision may occur if there is premature loading of the recently operated site, eg, the premature wearing of a denture, or a denture that is inadequately relieved and cushioned over the implant sites. Breakdown of the wound is particularly likely if there has been previous irradiation (Fig 10-2) or surgery (such as a visor osteotomy or the placement and removal of a subperiosteal implant) in the implant area. These factors all tend to impair the blood supply of the area.

Complications associated with abutment connection

It is sometimes difficult to judge with accuracy the desirable height of the abutments when they are placed. One may need to change the abutment later or use tempo-

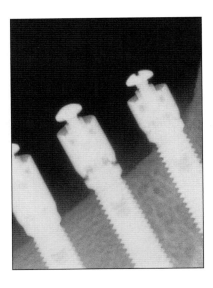

Fig 10-3 Note that one of the abutments in this radiograph is incompletely seated. This may lead to inflammatory problems and possible fistula formation. It should be corrected before treatment continues.

rary healing abutments until peri-implant soft tissues have healed and matured. The abutment cylinder must be accurately seated on the implant. Implant systems have internal, external, or tapered interfaces necessitating complete seating between the implant and the abutment. When these are incorrectly related or incompletely seated, soft tissue reactions such as hyperplasia and subsequent infection may result in fistula formation (Fig 10-3).

Cover screws placed on implants at the conclusion of stage 1 surgery (implant placement) also need to be completely and securely seated on top of the implant prior to soft tissue closure. On occasion, the tool used to place, seat, or remove the cover screw suffers fracture of its hexagonal tip, necessitating removal of the broken tip lodged in the cover screw.

Complications during restoration and maintenance

Abutment screws need to be properly preloaded with the correct torque prior to recording impressions toward prosthesis fabrication. Placement or removal of healing caps, or a patient's overtightening or inadvertent loosening of these caps between appointments, may result in loosening of abutment screws. It is critical to maintain a stable base onto which the prosthesis will ultimately rest. Therefore, it is prudent to check the status of abutment screws at each appointment during prosthesis fabrication. An implant framework that does not fit accurately will result in unfavorable distribution of load, which in turn may lead to compromise of the prosthetic components, screws, implant(s), or the prosthesis itself

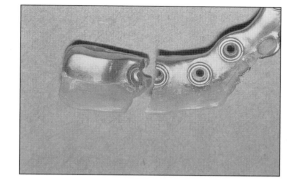

Fig 10-4 Fracture of the whole prosthesis, including the metal baseplate. The cross-sectional design of the baseplate casting is important, as is the length of the cantilever extension.

(Fig 10-4). Acrylic material used to provide the occlusal surface of the prosthesis may split and break off if it is not thick enough. Inadequate daily oral hygiene, particularly in peri-abutment sites that lack attached tissue, may result in inflammation and/or gingival hyperplasia.

A space created for hygiene access between the standard transmucosal abutment and the underside of the implant framework can result in an adjustment period for the patient when he or she is converting from a conventional tissue-borne prosthesis to an implant-supported prosthesis. In the mandible, this usually results in the creation of normal architecture as regards the patient's profile, ie, the area beneath the vermilion border of the lip becomes concave rather than convex as with a conventional complete denture flange, which plumps out the lower lip. In the maxillary arch, if the prosthesis is fabricated on transmucosal abutments, the space left between the ridge crest and the polished surface of the implant framework can result in the escape of air and saliva, leading to compromised

speech. Sometimes, this issue can be resolved by having a "gingival moll" or plumper fabricated of resilient resin (eg, Molloplast; Detax, Ettlingen, Germany) or heat-cured resin. The moll can be inserted and retained partly around the transmucosal abutments or be designed with various types of attachments to anchor it to the implant-supported prosthesis. Not infrequently, the patient's lip musculature seems to reorganize and adapt to this altered prosthesis contour such that initial concerns abate and cease to be an issue.

Serious complications

The placement of dental implants, like other oral surgical procedures, carries a small risk of serious complications, including fatality. Death from air embolism has resulted from the mistaken use of a coolant spray of compressed air and water used with internally irrigated drills.[2] This misguided practice has also caused serious surgical emphysema. Such tragedies are avoidable. Practitioners should not deviate

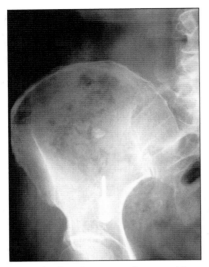

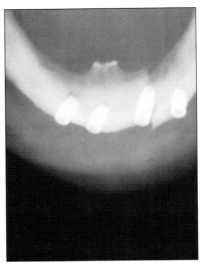

Fig 10-5 Radiograph showing a small screwdriver that was swallowed and became lodged in the patient's pelvic area; its progress was arrested at the ileocecal junction. The instrument was later removed successfully by fiberoptic colonoscopy.

Fig 10-6 Fracture of the mandible through the site of an endosseous cylindrical implant, shown on a radiograph.

from the manufacturers' recommendations regarding the use of equipment.

Life-threatening hemorrhage has been reported following instrumental perforation of the lingual cortex of the mandible during implant site preparation, with damage to small vessels in the adjacent floor of the mouth.[3,4] Bleeding may then progress into the soft tissues of the floor of the mouth, causing a threat to the patient's airway and necessitating emergency surgical treatment. Careful surgery, including exploration of lingual concavities, and postoperative patient supervision are needed to prevent this complication.

Many implant components are small, as are the instruments involved. When coated with saliva, a component may escape from the clinician's grip and fall into the oropharynx, where reflex swallowing may take the item out of sight almost immediately. This is a particular risk with a recumbent patient (Fig 10-5). The item may be ingested or, even worse, aspirated. If this should happen, the patient should be immediately placed in a head-down position and an attempt made to recover the lost component. If the component has gone too far, the patient should be transported to a hospital in a head-low position so that the appropriate endoscopy can be carried out.

Fracture of the atrophic mandible has been reported in several instances and certainly must have occurred in many unre-

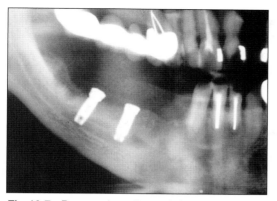

Fig 10-7a Panoramic radiograph indicating probable intrusion of implants into the inferior alveolar nerve canal.

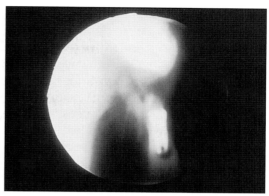

Fig 10-7b This tomogram confirms the penetration of an endosseous implant into the inferior alveolar canal. This resulted in loss of sensation in the mental nerve region.

ported cases (Fig 10-6).[5] This emphasizes the need for great care in patient evaluation, surgery, and aftercare. Patients with an atrophic mandible must be warned to take great care during the postoperative period. Treatment of a fractured atrophic mandible is never easy, but when the jawbone contains several recently placed, expensive implants occupying space that might otherwise be used for plates and screws, the situation is even more critical.

Damage to the inferior alveolar nerve due to misplaced implants has been reported (Figs 10-7a and 10-7b). Lingual perforation of the cortex resulting in impingement of the overlying periosteum can result from misangulation of the implant preparation site. This can lead to significant impingement on free nerve endings, resulting in symptoms that may necessitate removal or nonfunction of the implant ("putting it to sleep"). This indicates the need for detailed planning, including, in some cases, presurgi-

cal specialized radiographic assessment by computerized tomographic scans.

Complications associated with restorative treatment and maintenance

Among the complications that can occur once implant prosthodontic treatment is completed are loose or broken abutment screws or prosthetic retaining screws (gold screws); fracture of porcelain veneering material or resin denture teeth; cementation failures; and, with time, a need to reveneer the implant framework, eg, for resin-veneered, full-arch, implant-supported prostheses.

Complications between stage 1 and stage 2 surgery

With conventional two-stage surgery for osseointegrated implants, it is critical that adequate healing of the line of incision be complete before a tissue-supported treatment prosthesis is placed. Failure to do this puts the incision line at risk for breaking open, further delaying and/or compromising the healing process. Generally, adequate healing occurs for most patients between 7 and 14 days postoperative. There is a tendency for many patients to "push the envelope," wanting prosthesis placement to occur sooner than is recommended for healing. The second concern is overloading of the implants between stage 1 and 2. Adequate relief buccally, lingually, and crestally of at least 3 mm needs to be created such that enough resilient reline material can "cushion" the soft tissue overlying the implants during the healing period. When tissue overlying the implant(s) is particularly thin, a transitional prosthesis, even when adequately cushioned, can cause the cover screws to become exposed. In and of itself, exposure of cover screws does not lead to failure of osseointegration. It is recommended that the clinician advise the patient to maintain excellent hygiene around exposed cover screws so that infection is avoided. Since the introduction of the two-stage surgical approach for implant placement, some systems and clinicians have advocated a one-stage approach, which has proven to be successful relative to achieving osseointegration.

Diagnosis and clinical management of broken fixation screws at abutment or prosthesis levels can at times present significant challenges for the clinician. As mentioned previously, appropriate torque application to the screw fixation components is an essential prerequisite to eliminate or minimize the likelihood of this onerous situation. Patients frequently may or may not be aware that the unraveling of the system is occurring or has occurred. Some patients, however, are a good barometer for perceived sensations that indicate something has gone awry.

Loose or broken abutment screws in full-arch fixed implant prostheses often present with a soft tissue aberration, such as inflammation or fistula formation secondary to macromovement, that has resulted in percolation of microbacteria into the dead spaces in and around the abutment. Removal of the prosthesis often helps to diagnose the problem. Recovery of the residual threaded part of the abutment screw can, at times, be extremely challenging; several approaches have been used (some more successful than others). Rotation of an explorer tip or perioprobe over the top of the fractured component counterclockwise can gradually rotate out the broken component. Ultrasonic scalers also can assist in loosening and then allowing removal of the broken abutment screw. If the screw is particularly resistant to rotation, a small quarter-round bur or inverted cone bur can be used to "slot" the top of the broken component. In so doing, a custom-fabricated screwdriver made from a latch bur, such that it can engage the slot and rotate out the broken component, should be used. The latter approach must be done with extreme care so as to avoid damaging or scoring the internal threading of the implant. Some manufacturers of implants also have commercially available "easy outs" to recover broken threaded components as well as screw thread taps to retap the internal implant threads; both of these can be useful.

Fracture of the gold screw (prosthetic retaining screw) is less common, suggesting that the fulcrum or load distribution tends to be more inferior, ie, closer to the crest of bone. The change in design by manufacturers from a tapered-head gold screw design to a flat-head design also has led to a decrease in the incidence of gold screw fractures. This, combined with the recognized need to achieve the proper preload using appropriate torque control devices for securing retaining and abutment screws, has contributed significantly to a reduction in the incidence of screw loosening complications. Nonetheless, poor fit can lead to instances of gold screw loosening and/or fracture. It is prudent to preload screws at the time of prosthesis placement and then recheck the preload of the screws intermittently during the initial months of prosthesis use. Usually, at 1 month postplacement, the screws will have "stretched" to their elastic limit, necessitating retorquing to reestablish the recommended preload. Screws should then be spot-checked on quarterly recalls during the first year following prosthesis placement. At the 1-year follow-up, screws should again be checked and retorqued. If all is stable at the 1-year follow-up, the clinician should decide the frequency of rechecks for the life of the prosthesis. This monitoring should be titrated based on patient habits such as parafunctional activity, excessive loading from clenching, history of repeated tooth fracture, etc, which of necessity would mandate more frequent monitoring.

Fractured resin teeth

Patients can unknowingly overload the prosthesis, in part because of a lack of receptors normally found in the periodontal ligament surrounding natural teeth. Generally speaking, most patients do not overload implant prostheses, but when they do, the possibility of tooth fracture results. The most common tooth fracture is partial or incomplete. The options include direct and indirect replacement/repair. With direct repairs,

the missing part of the tooth can be restored by luting the broken piece, if available, with autopolymerizing clear or tooth-shade resin by first creating undercuts in the interface surfaces of the residual and broken piece. Alternatively, or if the broken piece was lost or swallowed, it can be repaired/replaced with light-cured, tooth-shade resin composite.

If the entire tooth has debonded and/or was lost, the prosthesis can be removed by disengagement of the gold screws, removal of the prosthesis, and then replacement with a tooth of the same shade and mold used in the fabrication of the prosthesis (it is important to keep a record of this in the patient's chart and/or lab box). As with conventional denture tooth replacement/repairs, the tooth can be indexed and then affixed to the prosthesis with repair acrylic.

Reveneer

With full-arch, implant-supported prostheses, tooth wear over time results in loss of the vertical dimension of occlusion. It is difficult to gauge when to recommend a reveneer of a patient's implant-supported prosthesis. Often, the incremental loss of vertical dimension of occlusion occurs very gradually and is not readily apparent to the patient. However, when a patient complains of loss of chewing function along with TMJ symptoms, reestablishing the vertical dimension of occlusion is the treatment of choice. Much in the same way that we cannot applaud with only one hand, a reveneer of the implant prosthesis necessitates restoration of the occlusal plane of the opposing arch, which in many cases is a maxillary complete denture, maxillary implant overdenture, or maxillary implant-supported prosthesis. The clinical and laboratory effort necessary to reveneer a full-arch, implant-supported prosthesis is roughly equivalent to the fabrication of complete dentures. The relative cost of this revision represents a fraction of the original treatment cost, and the restoration will likely continue to serve the patient for years to come.

Two points are very important, relative to informed consent and patient management: (1) Prior to entering into treatment, patients should be informed of the likely need for reveneering and its relative cost, and (2) the denture used for interim treatment between implant placement and prosthesis completion should be kept for use as a transitional treatment while reveneering procedures are being accomplished. Patients generally do not like to revert back to their transitional treatment after years of enjoying the benefits of an implant-supported prosthesis. Should the transitional treatment be misplaced, broken, etc, it is possible to fabricate a temporary transitional denture. This is accomplished by making an alginate impression of the existing implant-supported prosthesis, pouring a cast, and removing the implant prosthesis portion from the cast once recovered. The cast then approximates the residual ridge form with the abutments. Tooth-shade acrylic is then placed into the dentate portion of the alginate impression. The impression is placed into a pressure pot for 10 minutes. After the tooth-shade resin polymerizes, the newly created denture tooth portion of the treatment denture is recovered from the impression, trimmed, and reinserted into the impression. The impression is then filled with gingival-shade autopolymerizing resin, seated on the cast (which is coated with aluminum foil substitute), and then placed back into the pressure pot to generate a temporary prosthesis. After intraoral evaluation and adjustment

for seating of the transitional prosthesis, the prosthesis can be relined with resilient reline material over healing caps that are first placed on the transmucosal abutments, or over healing abutments if the prosthesis being reveneered is based at implant level.

The laboratory technician can burn off or cut off the worn teeth and clean and reopaque the framework. A wax rim is then placed on the framework, which can be adjusted clinically to the correct vertical dimension of occlusion. If the tooth mold, shade, and matrix were recorded and preserved, the teeth can be transferred from the matrix to the framework. Following try-in and verification of vertical dimension of occlusion, centric relation, esthetics, phonetics, lip support, etc, the prosthesis can then be processed in the laboratory. The reveneered prosthesis is then tried in, remounted, and the occlusion is refined; finally, the prosthesis is placed with appropriate preload of retaining screws.

Fractured porcelain

While the original tenets of implant prostheses advocated the use of resin teeth for their "shock-absorbing" considerations, many clinicians have opted to use porcelain veneering materials to restore implant prostheses. Needless to say, the rigidity of porcelain and the significant loads applied by patients to their implant treatments frequently lead to fracture of veneering materials. Depending on prosthesis design (ie, screw versus cement retention) the extent and location of the porcelain fracture can be managed by intraoral recontouring and polishing or prosthesis removal and stripping and reveneering the porcelain if the restoration is esthetically or functionally compromised. Porcelain repair materials can be used, but in most instances this has not proven to result in long-term resolution of compromise resulting from porcelain fracture. Currently, there is a trend in implant prosthodontics toward the use of cemented rather than screw-retained restorations. Some clinicians feel that cemented restorations offer several advantages relative to the esthetic and functional considerations. The caveat with this mindset is that, currently, there are no commercially available cements that are specifically formulated for a metal-to-metal interface. In light of the lack of a dedicated cement for implant restorations, two divergent approaches have been advocated: *(1)* use of a provisional or "soft" cement such as zinc oxide–eugenol with or without a modifier such as petroleum jelly, or *(2)* use of more durable "permanent" cements such as zinc phosphate, polycarboxylate, resin, or glass ionomer. However, the use of soft cements can result in debonding, often at inopportune times, which can lead to damage or loss of the prosthesis; and use of the "permanent" cements may mean that an otherwise acceptable prosthesis must be sectioned and removed to address abutment screw loosening. What is desperately lacking for the cement-retained implant prosthesis armamentarium is a reversible cement that could provide adequate retention and, when needed, the ability to reverse the retentive capability at will and in a controlled manner. While the concept in principle seems rudimentary, the development of such reversible cements is still wanting, not only for implant prostheses that are cement retained but also for conventional single-unit crowns and fixed partial dentures cemented on natural-tooth abutments.

Minimizing Complications

All implant systems have a history of complications.[6,7] These can usually be avoided by attention to detail throughout the whole period of patient care, from patient selection and treatment planning to the clinical and maintenance phases. Many complications can be avoided with thorough planning and attentive treatment. Careful follow-up often provides early detection of incipient complications. With reputable implant systems, the problems and complications that do occur are usually a result of deviation from recommended protocols and should diminish in frequency as the clinician gains experience. Complications deserve our most serious attention, not merely because of their effects on patients, but because the reputation of implant dentistry as a whole is at stake. Restorative dentists need to exercise the greatest care throughout the entire treatment period; small errors in planning or technique may produce greatly magnified effects.

References

1. Albrektsson T, Zarb GA, Worthington P, Eriksson AR. The long-term efficacy of currently used dental implants: A review and proposed criteria of success. Int J Oral Maxillofac Implants 1986;1: 11–25.
2. Davies JM, Campbell LA. Fatal air embolism during dental implant surgery: Report of three cases. Can J Anaesth 1990;37:112–121.
3. Mason ME, Triplett, RG, Alfonso WF. Life-threatening hemorrhage from placement of a dental implant. J Oral Maxillofac Surg 1990;48: 201–204.

4. Laboda G. Life-threatening hemorrhage after the placement of an endosseous implant: Report of a case. J Am Dent Assoc 1990;121:599–600.

5. Mason ME, Triplett RG, van Sickels JE, Parel SM. Mandibular fractures through endosseous cylinder implants: Report of cases and review. J Oral Maxillofac Surg 1990;8:311–317.

6. Worthington P, Bolender CL, Taylor TD. The Swedish system of osseointegrated implants: Problems and complications encountered during a 4-year trial period. Int J Oral Maxillofac Implants 1987;2:77–84.

7. Worthington P. Problems and complications with osseointegrated implants. In: Worthington P, Brånemark P-I (eds). Advanced Osseointegration Surgery: Applications in the Maxillofacial Region. Chicago: Quintessence, 1992:386–396.

chapter 11

Advanced Procedures with Implant Treatment

Philip Worthington, MD, BSc
Jeffrey E. Rubenstein, DMD, MS

The principal purpose of this book is to orient the dental student or novice in implant reconstruction to the role of osseointegration in the overall scheme of reconstructive measures. Consequently, emphasis has been placed on simpler situations and the safer, more predictable methods of rehabilitation. The student will soon become aware that at the cutting edge of clinical practice, some departures from these basic methods are being practiced. This is because more difficult clinical problems demand special measures. This chapter is intended to give the reader some introductory information about these more advanced techniques and the difficult situations where they may be appropriate. The student must understand that deviations from the orthodox protocol are almost always taken with some increased risk and hence are for the experienced clinician only.

Immediate Implants

While the standard two-stage approach advocated to achieve successful osseointegration remains the standard of care, innovations and modifications for this time-honored, proven approach have come on the horizon in the recent past. One such approach is the immediate placement of implants into extraction sites. Advocates for this approach feel they are able to preserve bony architecture, especially when placing implants in the "esthetic zone," ie, the anterior maxilla, where not only tooth replacement but also the development of optimal esthetics present significant challenges in the treatment of edentulous spaces with single-tooth implant restorations. Critics of immediate placement voice concerns about placing implants immediately into extraction sites because of possible compromise due to the fact that the extraction sites—especially those of periodontally compromised teeth—place the implants in foci of infection and also may not provide good bone-implant contact, since the tooth socket and implant shape may not be congruent. While early reports suggest successful outcomes of implant treatment with this approach, at the time of publication of this text, many mainstream practitioners view this approach as being a higher risk procedure versus the standard two-stage approach. Further long-term results are not yet available to substantiate claims of equivalent success/survival rates. The need for speed is often the driving force behind this "innovation." The merits of faster being better can be countered with the argument, "Why do we always have time to do it over but never have time to do it right?" Once again, the authors of this text would caution the neophyte implant practitioner to become well grounded in safe, predictable methods of implant treatment before embarking on higher risk procedures. Failure of implants, needless to say, is not a practice builder, leaving patients who have experienced failed implant treatment with little to show for their pursuit of tooth replacement other than lost time, emotional upheaval, and financial loss.

Immediate Loading

Early reports on immediate loading were limited to full-arch rehabilitation of the anterior mandible.[1] A 10-year follow-up report[2] suggested a reasonable level of implant success/survival with this approach. More recently, a number of reports on immediate or

early loading of implants for single-tooth and partial- and full-arch restorations have suggested results for the short term that are comparable to delayed implant placement/loading.[3–8] At the time of the publication of this text, it is suggested that inexperienced practitioners not embark on immediate placement/loading of implants until they are well grounded in more conventional and predictable implant treatment modalities. Evidence from long-term, well-controlled, longitudinal prospective clinical trials for much of what is done in regard to the use of implants is often lacking in the literature. Therefore, the treatment of patients with newer, less conventional approaches should be done with the utmost caution, especially as it relates to informed consent for patients seeking this type of care. Each failed implant treatment does little to foster positive reinforcement for implant therapy, and further, the ever-litigious public should serve as a barometer for the risk associated with providing more poorly scrutinized treatment procedures.

Brånemark Novum Concept

Dr P-I Brånemark's latest innovation and contribution to implant dentistry is the concept of "same-day teeth" (Novum, Nobel Biocare, Yorba Linda, CA). This approach employs a one-size-fits-all concept, using manufactured drilling templates and prefabricated implant frameworks to offer an assembly-line "erector set" approach for rehabilitation of the full-arch mandible and, more recently, the full-arch maxilla, with a fixed/detachable implant-supported prosthesis. The surgical expertise required to successfully and predictably treat a patient with the Novum approach involves significant surgical skill and experience. Patient selection also requires insight into which patients are suitable candidates for this approach. The current protocol calls for the placement of three implants in the mandible—one in the symphyseal region and one just anterior to the mental foramen bilaterally. The sites for these implants are predetermined with drilling templates and a specialized drilling protocol, which differs from that used for conventional implant placement. The Novum protocol calls for site preparations to maintain a precise interim-plant relationship. With such preparations, a prefabricated titanium "primary bar" can be placed immediately to splint the three implants, and on the same day of implant placement, a premachined framework that precisely fits the primary bar can be developed into a full-arch implant restoration. The prosthodontic, laboratory, and surgical teams need to be well coordinated in their mutual efforts to successfully facilitate treatment. A text authored by Dr Brånemark, outlining the treatment procedures and reporting on early results, serves as a resource for the reader to learn more about this treatment.[9]

Extreme Maxillary Atrophy

A patient with an edentulous maxilla that no can longer successfully support and retain a conventional complete denture presents a significant challenge as regards rehabilitation options. Typically, these patients present with radiographic evidence of little or no remaining bone volume for conventional implant placement. Often the posterior maxilla is resorbed to the floor of the sinus and/or the anterior maxilla is resorbed to the anterior nasal spine. Commensurate with the loss of bone volume is a loss of depth of the gingivobuccal sulcus. The edentulous patient with such compromise of the supporting structures of the maxilla represents one of the most significant challenges for rehabilitation with implant therapy. First and foremost, an effort to create a bone volume that will support an adequate number and distribution of implants is the cornerstone of the treatment plan for such cases. Bone grafting with autogenous bone, typically harvested from the iliac crest, is considered to be the "gold standard" against which alternative approaches are measured.[10] Grafting can take on a variety of approaches or combinations thereof. The bone graft can be placed as an onlay to the anterior maxilla and as an inlay into the nasal floor and/or maxillary sinus. Typically, patients with severe maxillary atrophy are best served by first augmenting the existing maxilla. In so doing, a bed is created into which implants can be placed and lost anatomy is restored. The base is established in such a way that the implant restoration will more correctly mirror that of the original anatomy associated with the natural teeth and supporting structures.

If ridge form is adequate but the vertical height of bone is deficient, eg, a large pneumatized maxillary sinus is present, then inlay bone grafting is the treatment of choice. Sinus elevation surgery to build bone height in the posterior maxilla has been shown to be an effective method for the facilitation of implant placement. Much has been researched, and many case series of sinus elevation surgery and implant placement have been published.[11] Generally speaking, sinus elevation surgery has been shown to improve the success/

survival potential for implant treatment in the posterior maxilla.[12] However, this type of implant therapy is considered to be tertiary care and is not a good place to begin developing experience with implant treatment.[13]

Alternatives to grafting the maxillary sinus have been developed. While not always a possibility, the pterygoid area has been shown to be a reliable site for implant placement.[14] First and foremost, an adequate volume of bone is a prerequisite for pterygoid implant placement. Further, the angle of placement creates a significant challenge for both the surgeon and restorative dentist, since the axial inclination, of necessity, orients the implant through the buccal aspect of the posterior maxilla. Seating of abutments and access to screws to secure prostheses present distinct challenges.

The zygomatic implant was introduced in the late 1990s by Dr Brånemark. This particular implant design uses implants that are much longer than average, on the order of 30 to 50 mm. The implant is placed palatally in the region of the zygomatic buttress (approximately the maxillary first or second molar area). The implant is then placed through the maxillary sinus, where there is no bone support, and then engages bone once again in the region of the zygoma. These implants generally are part of a base of support for a full-arch restoration or maxillary implant overdenture. Additional implants of various lengths must be placed in the anterior maxilla. The patient with deficient bone in the posterior maxilla thus avoids the need to graft this area for implant placement.[10] The limited evidence available thus far suggests an equivalent success rate in comparison to conventional implant treatments.

Distraction Osteogenesis

The technique of distraction osteogenesis was originally developed as a means of elongating long bones, such as those of the leg. It involved a partial transsection of the bone (at least a cut through the cortex, or corticotomy), following which the two segments were mechanically and slowly distracted from one another using pins and an external framework. As the segments were separated, healing callus was laid down at the plane of section, in the gap, and this was transformed into mature bone over time. Initially after the section, a latent period is allowed while callus begins to form; then distraction is effected slowly—perhaps 1 mm each day. In this way, bones can be lengthened significantly. Once the distraction is completed, there must be a period of stabilization so that the newly formed bone, which is at first rather plastic, can consolidate and mature.

This technique has many applications in the maxillofacial region as an alternative to more traditional procedures of orthognathic surgery; in the field of implant reconstruction it can, for example, be used in the form of vertical alveolar distraction to remedy an alveolar process that is deficient in height. This is just one example of how distraction osteogenesis can serve to improve a potential implant site. For further discussion, the reader is referred to Jensen's *Alveolar Distraction Osteogenesis*.[15]

Guided Bone Regeneration

If a void exists alongside stable bone, the clinician may consider improving a potential implant site by onlay bone grafting, but an alternative to be considered is the technique of *guided bone regeneration*. In this method, bone is induced to form in the void, as opposed to the space being filled with connective tissue of a lower order of differentiation. The void may be covered by a special type of membrane that excludes the ingrowth of simpler fibrous tissue elements but allows bone to grow into the space. To accelerate this process, the void may be filled with bone grafting material, eg, particulate spongy bone. When covered by a membrane, this graft then consolidates and matures, rather than being resorbed and replaced by fibrous tissue. This process, whereby less desirable connective tissue components are selectively excluded but the development of bone-forming tissue is allowed, is dependent on the limited permeability of the membrane. Currently, both resorbable and nonresorbable types of membranes are available. This can be a very valuable means of improving an implant site. For more detailed discussion, the reader is referred to *Guided Bone Regeneration in Implant Dentistry*, edited by Buser et al.[16]

Implants in Orthodontic Treatment

For successful orthodontic movement of teeth, one essential is a healthy and complete periodontium, ie, a periodontal ligament and alveolar bone. The next essential for teeth to move under orthodontic forces is a fixed point of anchorage from which, or to which, the orthodontic "push" or "pull" can act. Given these essentials, tooth movement can be accomplished by the processes of bone remodeling, resorption, and deposi-

tion. Osseointegrated implants can provide this anchorage, since they do not move through bone under orthodontic forces; there is no periodontal ligament around an implant, hence, the implant anchorage units remain firm. This special and important application of osseointegration is discussed in detail in Higuchi's *Orthodontic Applications of Osseointegrated Implants*.[17]

Cancer Reconstruction

There is no population better served by the introduction of osseointegration than that of the patient requiring oral rehabilitation following ablative surgery to eradicate oral carcinoma. Patients requiring these rehabilitative services are seldom managed in general practice but are a focus of activity in major teaching institutions and medical centers worldwide. These patients range in age from the very young to the very old. More commonly, however, the older adult is the recipient of this type of care. The complexity of managing rehabilitative efforts for this group of patients cannot be covered in great detail in this text. Each case is a unique entity, and the clinician therefore requires a great deal of ingenuity to develop the appropriate treatment regimen that will restore function to severely compromised oral anatomy. Ablation, reconstruction, and rehabilitation require a team effort by many specialists. In today's approach to such rehabilitation, a microvascular free flap harvested from the fibula, scapula, ilium, or radius is often used to reconstruct missing parts of the maxilla and/or mandible. Soft tissue vascularized grafts, such as the radial forearm flap and rectus abdominus flap, are used to reconstruct soft tissue anatomy such as the tongue and soft palate.

Once the graft has matured and the patient is deemed ready for oral rehabilitation, treatment prostheses are developed to assist in planning where implants can be placed to adequately support the anticipated prosthesis(es). The mere replacement of missing dentition does not in and of itself rehabilitate this type of patient. Rather, it is the development of the prosthesis(es) in such a way that coordinates the remaining soft tissues such that function is maximized. In many instances the "rehabilitation" of necessity offers limited functional improvement. In large measure, this is often not the fault of the completed prosthesis but rather a function of the remaining soft tissues such as the lips, the tongue, the soft palate, the muscles, and the innervation associated with these structures. It is often difficult to measure the functional outcome for a patient so compromised, and on an individual basis, it is difficult to measure the benefit of the rehabilitation effort. The saving grace associated with these rehabilitation attempts often is the incredible will of the patient, whose desire to be restored to function and be made whole is the uncontrolled variable that facilitates improved function to a larger degree than the treatment provided.

In today's treatment protocols for the management of head and neck cancer, a variety of modalities have expanded the armamentarium beyond the standard approach of surgical excision with or without pre- or postoperative radiotherapy. More commonly today, especially for those patients diagnosed with advanced neoplastic disease, adjunctive or concomitant chemotherapy used in conjunction with radiotherapy has shown some promise in reducing tumor volume and maintaining local control of the

disease. More aggressive radiotherapeutic regimens—high-energy photons, electrons, neutrons, and protons—have also become additions to the radiotherapy armamentarium to provide more comprehensive treatment of tumor and nodal sites, thereby improving dose distribution. Intraoperative treatment schemes such as gamma knife and stereotactic radiotherapy are also commonly used. The compromised tissue that remains and now is called upon to support prostheses and withstand functional loading from those prostheses creates an inherent conundrum, which puts the clinician in a quandary and the patient at risk for complications. It is our duty to "do no harm" in the provision of oral rehabilitative efforts; since we are not armed with a crystal ball telling us which patient will or will not be able to tolerate oral rehabilitative efforts, we must proceed with the utmost caution.

In the past, the patient with a compromised mandible following tumor ablation was commonly left with a discontinuity defect if the lesion was located in the posterior mandible; a compromised residual ridge if the tumor involved the alveolus minimally; or an "Andy Gump" defect (ie, a defect in which the mandible is severely retrognathic to the extent that the patient appears to have "no chin," as is seen in the cartoon character Andy Gump) if bone involvement occurred in the anterior mandible, requiring resection. Any of these defects of the mandible and adjacent soft tissue resulted in significant functional compromise in speech, swallowing, and mastication. The restoration of continuity of the mandible with currently available grafting techniques has given back to these patients missing oral structures and function that were only dreams of earlier patients and their clinicians. The treatment of choice for patients with restored continuity of the mandible is the implant-supported prosthesis.

Patients with an irradiated jaw

Radiation impairs the blood supply to the irradiated jaw, and that in turn implies impaired healing capacity. When the radiation dose exceeds 5,000 cGy we recommend that pre-implant treatment with hyperbaric oxygen be made part of the treatment protocol, especially in the mandible. Hyperbaric oxygen treatment has many features, but one is the encouragement of neoangiogenesis in the tissues, and this goes a long way to counteracting the relative ischemia that results from radiation therapy. While this issue of the use of hyperbaric oxygen remains a topic of debate, certain facts are well supported in the literature:

1. When implants are placed into irradiated bone, there is less bone formed at the interface.
2. The bone formed at the interface is of lesser quality.
3. Removal force values are lower.
4. Overall success rates for these implants are lower, especially for some sites.
5. There is some evidence of continuing implant loss over time.
6. There are risks of nonintegration, less ideal integration, less durable integration, soft tissue necrosis, and osteoradionecrosis.

It is true that implant surgery can be successful in irradiated tissues that do not receive hyperbaric oxygen—but seemingly less predictably. Proponents of hyperbaric oxygen take the view that the clinician is obligated to give the patient the highest degree of integration possible, rather than practice on the basis of what we can "get away with."

Discontinuity defects

Many patients with tumors involving the posterior lateral border of the tongue or the floor of the mouth, or with alveolar ridge tumors involving the posterior aspect of the mandible, have surgical intervention resulting in loss of continuity of the mandible. Currently, these defects are being reconstructed with various types of nonvascularized and vascularized bone grafting procedures. However, some patients are left with discontinuity defects, ie, a residual mandible with only one remaining functioning condyle. If a patient with such a discontinuity defect is also edentulous, rehabilitation with a mandibular conventional tissue-borne resection denture has a limited, if not abysmal, prognosis for functional rehabilitation. The use of implants to either retain or support a replacement dentition promises improved oral function. However, it should be noted that restoring continuity to the mandible offers substantially greater functional improvement in conjunction with implant rehabilitation. As mentioned previously, surgical ablation with postoperative radiotherapy further complicates rehabilitation treatment protocols, and generally speaking, a fixed detachable implant-supported prosthesis is preferable to a removable implant overdenture prosthesis.

Reconstruction After Trauma

Many trauma victims can benefit from implant reconstruction. This includes patients who have lost teeth and perhaps alveolar bone in a sporting accident, a motor vehicle accident, an industrial accident, or as the result of a gunshot wound. In common with the cancer patient, there may be tissue loss (both hard and soft), scarring, and/or denervation (both sensory and motor). Each case is unique and demands ingenuity in devising the best form of reconstruction/rehabilitation. The steps may well include grafting of tissue, implant placement, and prosthesis fabrication. Fixed prostheses are generally preferable to removable prostheses.

Reconstruction of Developmental Anomalies

Defects in development may range from the congenitally missing single tooth through total anodontia, and from cleft lip and palate through multiple craniofacial syndromes, such as craniofacial dysostosis, acrocephalosyndactyly (Apert syndrome), and notably ectodermal dysplasia. All such cases need the coordinated efforts of the reconstructive and rehabilitative teams, and implants can play a fundamental role in treatment. Because of considerations of growth and development, the timing of implant placement may be critical.

Craniofacial Prostheses

One of the more recent developments in the realm of implant treatment is the introduction of a modified design known as the craniofacial implant.[18] These implants are designed to be used to assist in retaining prostheses made of medical-grade, tissue-colored silicone to restore missing anatomic structures. Prior to the introduction of craniofacial implants, patients requiring these types of replacements retained their auricular, nasal, orbital, or multisite prostheses with a variety of adhesives to affix them to the skin. Alternatively, where facial defects presented with soft tissue undercuts, eg, an orbital exenteration, these offered the potential to mechanically retain the prosthesis. This approach met with some limited success in improving retention, when tolerated by the patient's tissues.

Craniofacial implants have been used in the United States since 1988.[19] The missing auricle is the most frequent application, followed by nasal, then orbital, then midface or combinations of anatomic sites. Typically, an auricular prosthesis can be retained with the placement of two craniofacial implants placed approximately 18 to 20 mm posterior to the auricular canal, if present. A nasal prosthesis also can be adequately retained with two implants, which are typically placed in the lateral alar regions. For an orbital prosthesis, the number of implants placed is largely dictated by the available bone. If only the superior and lateral portions of the orbital rim are intact, then three or perhaps four implants are placed. If the superior, lateral, and inferior portions of the orbital rim are intact, typically three well-distributed implants can be used to individually retain a prosthesis with magnetic retention. If a wide distribution of implants cannot be obtained, the implants that are able to be placed are typically splinted to facilitate cantilevering the bar into areas where there is adequate retention for the prosthesis.

With increasing experience, clinicians and technicians have collaborated to develop improved designs for retaining facial prostheses using a variety of attachments, including resilient attachments and magnets. Clearly, retention of the prosthesis with an implant approach offers significant advantages to that of adhesive-retained prostheses. Patient acceptance of facial prostheses in large measure is predicated on the provision of reliable and predictable retention. The craniofacial implant offers a reliable mechanism for retaining facial prostheses; however, the material of which facial prostheses are fabricated has a limited length of service, necessitating the need for remakes annually or nearly annually, depending in large measure on patient factors such as quality of maintenance and environmental factors such as the amount of sun exposure, particulate matter, and chemical pollutants. The next challenge for the implant-retained facial prosthesis is to match the longevity of the prosthesis with that of the long-term survival of the implants used to retain them.

A craniofacial implant has also been employed to assist individuals with sensory-neural auditory compromise; the implant is used along with a specially designed abutment that retains a transmitter to amplify sound for bone conduction hearing assistance. This approach is known as the bone-anchored hearing aid (BAHA). The size of the transmitter has become smaller since its initial introduction. Patients treated with the BAHA have clearly documented improvement in hearing.

Orthopedic Applications

A number of exciting expanded applications of osseointegrated technology have been developed by Dr Brånemark. Among these developments are specially designed implants for joint, limb, and digit replacement.

The same basic tenets for establishing a bone-to-implant connection serve as the cornerstone for successful treatment of these very challenging anatomic compromises. Stemming from these types of treatments is a new term that Dr Brånemark calls *osseoperception*, whereby the anatomic site replaced with this approach not only is provided with a prosthesis but, via the connection to the implant, receives a perceived neurosensory input that mimics in part normal sensation. For example, a patient with a mid-femur amputation rehabilitated with an implant-retained leg prosthesis can discern through the implant the type of surface the limb is resting on. In other words, the patient can sense whether the limb is supporting the patient's weight on, eg, a wood floor, concrete sidewalk, lawn, or carpet. An implant-retained thumb prosthesis can be used by the patient to hold a pen and even harvest an egg from a chicken coop without breaking the shell.

As technologic advances continue, the range of applications surely will continue to expand and provide significant improvements for examples of anatomic compromise. This will not be limited to oral rehabilitation, but functional improvement will be available for a wide range of rehabilitation needs.

References

1. Schnitman PA, Wohrle PS, Rubenstein JE. Immediate fixed interim prostheses supported by two-stage threaded implants. Methodology and results. J Oral Implantol 1990;16:96–105.
2. Schnitman PA, Wohrle PS, Rubenstein JE, DaSilva JD, Wang N-H. Ten-year results of Brånemark implants immediately loaded with fixed prostheses at implant placement. Int J Oral Maxillofac Implants 1997;12:495–503.

3. Ericsson I, Nilson H, Lindh T, Nilner K, Randow K. Immediate functional loading of Brånemark single tooth implants. An 18 months' clinical pilot follow-up study. Clin Oral Implants Res 2000;11: 26–33.

4. Kan JYK, Rungcharassaeng K, Lozada JL. Immediate placement and provisionalization of maxillary single implants: 1-year prospective study. Int J Oral Maxillofac Implants 2003;18:31–39.

5. Wohrle P. Single-tooth replacement in the aesthetic zone with immediate provisionalization: Fourteen consecutive case reports. Pract Periodontics Aesthet Dent 1998;10:1107–1114.

6. Cooper L, Felton D, Kugelberg C, et al. A multicenter 12-month evaluation of single-tooth implants restored 3 weeks after 1-stage surgery. Int J Oral Maxillofac Implants 2001;16:182–192.

7. Rocci A, Matignoni M, Gottlow J. Immediate loading of Brånemark system TiUnite and machined-surface implants in the posterior mandible: A randomized open-ended clinical trial. Clin Implant Dent Relat Res 2003;5(suppl 1):57–62.

8. Balshi TJ, Wolfinger GJ. Immediate loading of Brånemark implants in edentulous mandibles. A preliminary report. Implant Dent 1997;6:83–88.

9. Brånemark P-I, Svensson B (eds). The Brånemark Novum Protocol for Same-Day Teeth: A Global Perspective. Chicago: Quintessence, 2001.

10. Brånemark P-I, Grondahl K, Worthington P. Osseointegration and Autogenous Onlay Bone Grafts. Chicago: Quintessence, 2001.

11. Collins T, Small S, Shepherd N, Busser D, Parel S. Sinus floor elevation and the status of membranes. Int J Oral Maxillofac Implants 1994;9 (suppl):85–105.

12. Jensen OT, Shulman LB, Block MS, Iacono VJ. Report of the Sinus Consensus Conference of 1996. Int J Oral Maxillofac Implants 1998;13(suppl): 11–45.

13. Jensen OT (ed). The Sinus Bone Graft. Chicago: Quintessence, 1999.

14. Tulasne JF. Osseointegrated fixtures in the pterygoid region. In: Worthington P, Brånemark P-I (eds). Advanced Osseointegration Surgery: Applications in the Maxillofacial Region. Chicago: Quintessence, 1992:182–188.

15. Jensen OT (ed). Alveolar Distraction Osteogenesis. Chicago: Quintessence, 2002.

16. Buser D, Dahlin C, Schenk RK (eds). Guided Bone Regeneration in Implant Dentistry. Chicago: Quintessence, 1994.

17. Higuchi K (ed). Orthodontic Applications of Osseointegrated Implants. Chicago: Quintessence, 2000.

18. Tjellstrom A. Osseointegrated implants for the replacement of absent or defective ears. Clin Plast Surg 1990;17:355-366.

19. Brånemark P-I, Tolman DE (eds). Osseointegration in Craniofacial Reconstruction. Chicago: Quintessence, 1998.

chapter 12

Conclusion

Philip Worthington, MD, BSc

It will soon be 40 years since Professor Brånemark demonstrated the phenomenon of osseointegration in a clinical situation. His first oral implants were placed in a patient in 1965; since then, much experience has been gained worldwide in both clinical practice and research. Given certain requirements, the successful biologic integration of a titanium component into living bone was shown to be achievable, reproducible, and predictable. Those requirements included prudent patient selection, the use of biocompatible materials, adherence to a strict surgical protocol, skilled prosthodontic care, and diligent maintenance. Efforts have been made over the years to bend the rules, to "push the envelope," and some of these efforts have been successful. Not all have been well advised. We may now look back over these many years and review the developments that have taken place.

The essentials of surgical placement remain the same. However, under certain circumstances, variations in timing can be tolerated: for example, single-stage placement may sometimes justifiably replace the conventional two-stage surgery. There are variations in width and length and overall shape of surgical components, eg, threaded or nonthreaded, cylindrical or tapered. Variations have been tried in the surface preparation of implants and in coatings. Changes have been made in implant site preparation, going beyond onlay bone grafting to the use of bone substitutes, guided bone regeneration, distraction osteogenesis, the use of tissue sealants, and most recently bone morphogenetic proteins. The topographic placement of implants—their spacing, angulation, and alignment—has been aided by computer programs. Furthermore, implants have been developed for special sites such as the pterygoid region and the zygomatic bone.

However, it was always foreseeable that the greatest changes would come in the field of restorative treatment. Not only have there been great developments in the range and design of available abutments but also in the materials of which they are made.

Whereas most early restorations were retrievable (screw-retained), many are now cemented. Fundamental changes have been attempted in the timing of prosthodontic treatment, with trials of immediate loading as opposed to traditional delayed loading.

The range of application of osseointegration has also been extended. Initially the most common application was in the field of dental implants to replace missing teeth; now implants are used to assist orthodontic tooth movement. Outside the oral cavity, the same technology is used in craniofacial implants to support prostheses for the replacement of the external ear, the nose, the orbit and its contents, and occasionally large segments of the face. The use of bone-anchored hearing aids is rapidly expanding. In orthopedics, osseointegration has been used successfully for joint replacement surgery and for the attachment of missing digits and limb amputation prostheses.

Even a cursory review of the wide range of applications of osseointegration reveals how many patients have derived enormous benefit from the discovery of this biologic phenomenon. Patients and clinicians alike owe a great debt to those who discovered osseointegration and those who worked patiently and persistently to refine its applications. We do well to remember, however, that osseointegration surgery is very technique sensitive, and even small changes in the practical steps may have profound variations in the end results.

Central to the philosophy underlying osseointegration is a respect for biology. The aim is to harness and use the body's capacity for healing and repair—to use it to our advantage, not to abuse it. Beginners should appreciate that many of the current developments in clinical practice still await the results of long-term trials. They would be wise to use well-tried, conventional strategies rather than adopt the latest trend in accelerated treatment. Remember the old adage: *Be not the first by whom the new is tried, nor yet the last to cast the old aside.*

Index